Virtual Clinical Excursions—General Hospital

for

Harkreader and Hogan:
Fundamentals of Nursing:
Caring and Clinical Judgment
2nd Edition

Virtual Clinical Excursions—General Hospital

for

Harkreader and Hogan:
Fundamentals of Nursing:
Caring and Clinical Judgment
2nd Edition

prepared by

Helen Harkreader, PhD, RN
Professor
Austin Community College
Austin, Texas

Marita T. Peppard, RN, ND, MS
Professor
Austin Community College
Austin, Texas

Virtual Clinical Excursions Author and Software Design

Jay Shiro Tashiro, PhD, RN
Director of Systems Design
Wolfsong Informatics
Tucson, Arizona

Ellen Sullins, PhD
Director of Research
Wolfsong Informatics
Tucson, Arizona

Gina Long, RN, DNSc
Assistant Professor, Department of Nursing
College of Health Professions
Northern Arizona University
Flagstaff, Arizona

Software Development

Michael Kelly
Developer and Programmer
Michael M. Kelly and Associates
Flagstaff, Arizona

SAUNDERS
An Imprint of Elsevier Science
Philadelphia   London   New York   St. Louis   Sydney   Toronto

SAUNDERS, INC.

11830 Westline Industrial Drive
St. Louis, Missouri 63146

Notice

Pharmacology is an ever-changing field. Standard safety precautions must be followed, but as new research and clinical experience broaden our knowledge, changes in treatment and drug therapy may become necessary or appropriate. Readers are advised to check the most current product information provided by the manufacturer of each drug to be administered to verify the recommended dose, the method and duration of administration, and contraindications. It is the responsibility of the licensed prescriber, relying on experience and knowledge of the patient, to determine dosages and the best treatment for each individual patient. Neither the publisher nor the editor assumes any liability for any injury and/or damage to persons or property arising from this publication.

The Publisher

First Edition 2004.

Executive Vice President, Nursing & Health Professions: Sally Schrefer
Editor, Nursing: Tom Wilhelm
Senior Developmental Editor: Jeff Downing
Project Manager: Gayle May
Designer: Wordbench
Cover Art: Jyotika Schrof

Printed in the United States of America

Last digit is the print number: 9   8   7   6   5   4   3   2   1

Workbook
prepared by

Helen Harkreader, PhD, RN
Professor
Austin Community College
Austin, Texas

Marita T. Peppard, RN, ND, MS
Professor
Austin Community College
Austin, Texas

Textbook

Helen Harkreader, PhD, RN
Professor
Austin Community College
Austin, Texas

Mary Ann Hogan, RN, CS, MSN
Clinical Assistant Professor
School of Nursing
University of Massachusetts
Amherst, Massachusetts

Contents

Table of Contents—Harkreader and Hogan: Fundamentals of Nursing: Caring and Clinical Judgment 2nd edition

Getting Started

GETTING SET UP

■ MINIMUM SYSTEM REQUIREMENTS

Virtual Clinical Excursions—General Hospital is a hybrid CD, so it runs on both Macintosh and Windows platforms. To use *Virtual Clinical Excursions—General Hospital*, you will need one of the following systems:

- **Windows™**

  Windows XP, 2000, 98, 95, NT 4.0
  IBM-compatible computer
  Pentium II processor (or equivalent)
  300 MHz
  96 MB (minimum) of RAM
  800 × 600 screen size
  Thousands of colors
  100 MB hard drive space
  12× CD-ROM drive
  Soundblaster 16 soundcard compatibility
  Stereo speakers or headphones

- **Macintosh®**

  MAC OS 9.04
  Apple Power PC G3
  300 MHz
  96 MB (minimum) of RAM
  800 × 600 screen size
  Thousands of colors
  100 MB hard drive space
  12× CD-ROM drive
  Stereo speakers or headphones

Note: *Virtual Clinical Excursions—General Hospital* is not designed to function at a 256-color depth. You may need to go to the Control Panel and change the Display settings. Instructions on adjusting these settings may be found in the How to Adjust Your Monitor's Settings on p. 2 of this workbook.

1

■ **INSTALLING** *VIRTUAL CLINICAL EXCURSIONS—GENERAL HOSPITAL*

- **Windows™**

  1. Start Microsoft Windows and insert *Virtual Clinical Excursions—General Hospital* **Disk 1** in the CD-ROM drive.
  2. Click the **Start** button on the taskbar and select the **Run** option.
  3. Type d:\Windows 95 setup.exe or d:\Windows 98-XP setup.exe (depending on your operating system—where "d:\" is your CD-ROM drive) and press **OK**.
  4. Follow the on-screen instructions for installation.
  5. Remove *Virtual Clinical Excursions—General Hospital* **Disk 1** from your CD-ROM drive.
  6. Restart your computer.

- **Macintosh®**

  1. Insert *Virtual Clinical Excursions—General Hospital* **Disk 1** in the CD-ROM drive. The disk icon will appear on your desktop.
  2. Double-click on the disk icon.
  3. Double-click on the icon that reads **Install Virtual Clinical Excursions**.
  4. Follow the on-screen instructions for installation.
  5. Remove *Virtual Clinical Excursions—General Hospital* **Disk 1** from your CD-ROM drive.
  6. Restart your computer.

■ **HOW TO ADJUST YOUR MONITOR'S SETTINGS (WINDOWS™ ONLY)**

- **Windows 95/98/SE/ME/2000**

  1. Click the **Start** button and go to **Settings** on the pop-up menu. Click on **Control Panel**.
  2. When the Control Panel window opens, double-click on the **Display** icon.
  3. You will now be presented with the Display Properties window. Click on the **Settings** tab (on the right). Below the image of the monitor, you will see on the left the **Color** palette. (You should change this to **High Color [16 bit]** by selecting it from the drop-down menu. You will need to restart your computer to do this.) On the right is the desktop area. Left-click and hold down on the slider button and move it to 800 by 600 pixels. Now click **OK**.
  4. Windows will ask you to confirm the change; click **OK**. Your screen will resize and Windows will again ask you whether you want to keep these new settings. Click **Yes**.

- **Windows XP**

  1. Click the **Start** button; then click **Control Panel** on the pop-up menu.
  2. Click **Display**. If Display does not appear, click **Switch to Classic View**; then click on **Display** icon.
  3. From the Display Properties dialog box, select the **Settings** tab.
  4. Under Screen Resolution, click and drag the sliding bar to adjust the desktop size to 800 x 600 pixels.
  5. Under Color Quality, choose **High** or **Highest**.
  6. Click **Apply**. If you approve of the new settings, click **Yes**.

■ HOW TO ACCESS PATIENTS

Unlike previous VCE products that presented all of the patients on one disk, *Virtual Clinical Excursions—General Hospital* includes patients on both disks. Both of the patients on the Pediatric Floor (Floor 3) are found on Disk 1, which you used to install the program. The remaining patients—including three patients in the Medical-Surgical-Telemetry Unit (Floor 6), one patient in the Intensive Care Unit (Floor 5), and one patient who spends time in the Medical-Surgical-Telemetry Unit (Floor 6) and in the Surgery Department (Floor 4)—are located on Disk 2. When you want to work with any of the seven patients in the virtual hospital, follow these steps:

- **Windows™**

    1. Insert the *Virtual Clinical Excursions—General Hospital* disk that contains the patient you want to work with into your CD-ROM drive.
    2. Double-click on the icon **Shortcut to Virtual Clinical Excursions**, which can be found on your desktop. This will load and run the program.

- **Macintosh®**

    1. Insert the *Virtual Clinical Excursions—General Hospital* disk that contains the patient you want to work with into your CD-ROM drive.
    2. Double-click on the icon **Shortcut to Virtual Clinical Excursions**, which can be found on your desktop. This will load and run the program.

■ QUALITY OF VISUALS, SPEED, AND COMMON PROBLEMS

Virtual Clinical Excursions—General Hospital uses the Apple QuickTime media layer system. This includes QuickTime Video and QuickTime VR Video, which allow for high-quality graphics and digital video. The graphics seen in the *Virtual Clinical Excursions—Medical-Surgical* courseware should be of high quality with rich color. If the movies and graphics appear blocky or grainy, check to see whether your video card is set to "thousands of colors."

Note: Virtual Clinical Excursions—General Hospital is not designed to function at a 256-color depth. To adjust your monitor's settings, see instructions on p. 2.

The system should respond quickly and smoothly. In particular, you should not see any jerky motions or experience unusual delays as you move through the virtual hospital settings, interact with patients, or access information resources. If you notice slow, jerky, or delayed software responses, it may mean that your particular system requires additional RAM, your processor does not meet the basic requirements, or your hard drive is full or too fragmented. If the videos appear banded or subject to "breakup," you may need to find an updated video driver for the computer's video card. Please consult the manufacturer of the video card or computer for additional video drivers for your machine.

If you are experiencing misplacement of text or cursors in the Electronic Patient Record (EPR), it is likely that your computer operating system has enabled font smoothing. Please turn font smoothing off by following these instructions:

- **Windows™**

    From the Control Panel window click on **Display** and then select the **Appearance** tab. Click on **Effects** and make sure the box next to "Smooth Edges of Screen Fonts" option is unselected.

- **Macintosh®**

    From the desktop, click on the **Apple** icon in the upper left corner. From the drop-down menu, select **Control Panel**; then select **Appearance**. Click on the **Fonts** tab and make sure the selection box next to "Smooth all fonts on screen" is unselected.

Virtual Clinical Excursions—General Hospital uses Adobe Acrobat Reader version 5 to display information in certain places in the simulation. If you cannot see any information when accessing the Charts, Medication Administration Record (MAR), or Kardex, it is likely that Adobe Acrobat Reader was not installed properly when you installed *Virtual Clinical Excursions—General Hospital*. To remedy this, you can manually install Acrobat Reader from the *Virtual Clinical Excursions—General Hospital* **Disk 1**. Double-click the **Adobe Acrobat Reader** installer (ar505enu.exe) on the disk and follow the on-screen instructions. Once the installer has finished installing Acrobat Reader, restart your computer and then resume your use of *Virtual Clinical Excursions—General Hospital*.

■ TECHNICAL SUPPORT

Technical support for this product is available at no charge by calling the Technical Support Hotline between 9 a.m. and 5 p.m. (Central Time), Monday through Friday. Inside the United States, call 1-800-692-9010. Outside the United States, call 314-872-8370.

Trademarks: Windows™ is a registered trademark.

A QUICK TOUR

Welcome to *Virtual Clinical Excursions—General Hospital*, a virtual hospital setting in which you can work with seven patient simulations and also learn to access and evaluate the health information resources that are essential for high-quality patient care.

The virtual hospital, **Canyon View Regional Medical Center**, is a multistory teaching hospital with a Well-Child Clinic, Pediatric Floor, Surgery Department, Intensive Care Unit, and a Medical-Surgical Floor with a Telemetry Unit. You will have access to the adult patients in the Intensive Care Unit and on the Medical-Surgical Floor. One patient will also spend time in the Surgery Department, where you can follow her through a perioperative experience.

Although each floor plan in the medical center is different, each is based on a realistic hospital architecture modeled from a composite of several hospital settings. All floors have:

- A Nurses' Station
- Patients, seen either in examination areas or in their inpatient rooms
- Patient records, including a Chart, Kardex plan of care, Medication Administration Record, and Electronic Patient Record accessed through a simulated computerized system.

■ BEFORE YOU START

When you use *Virtual Clinical Excursions—General Hospital*, make sure you have your textbook nearby to consult topic areas as needed. Also make sure that you have both disks to run the simulations. If you have not already installed your *VCE—General Hospital* software, do so now by following the steps outlined in **Getting Set Up** at the beginning of this workbook.

■ ENTERING THE HOSPITAL AND SELECTING A CLINICAL ROTATION

To begin your tour of Canyon View Regional Medical Center, insert your *Virtual Clinical Excursions—General Hospital* Disk 2 and double-click on the desktop icon **Shortcut to VCE—General Hospital**. Wait for the hospital entrance screen to appear (see below). This is your signal that the program is ready to run. Your first task is to get to the unit where you will be caring for patients and to let someone know when you arrive at the unit. As in any multistory hospital, you will enter the hospital lobby area, take an elevator to your assigned unit, and sign in at the Nurses' Station.

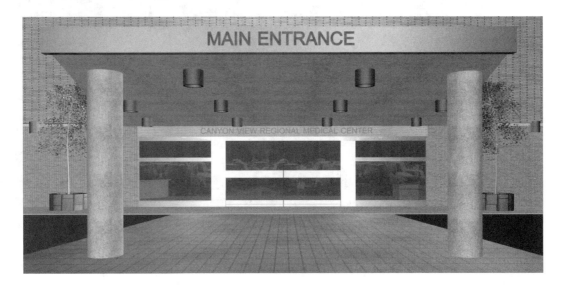

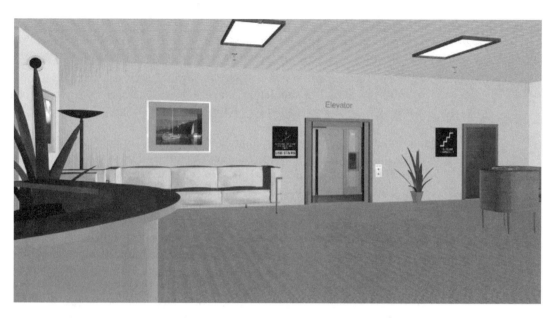

Let's practice getting to your unit in Canyon View Regional Medical Center by following this sequence:

- Click on the hospital entrance door and you will find yourself in the hospital lobby on the first floor (see above).
- Across the lobby, you will see an elevator with a blinking red light. Click on the open doorway and you will be transported into the elevator (see below).
- Now click on the panel on the right side of the doorway. The panel will expand to reveal buttons that allow you to go to the other floors of the hospital (see p. 7).
- Slowly run your cursor across the buttons to familiarize yourself with the different floors and units of the hospital.

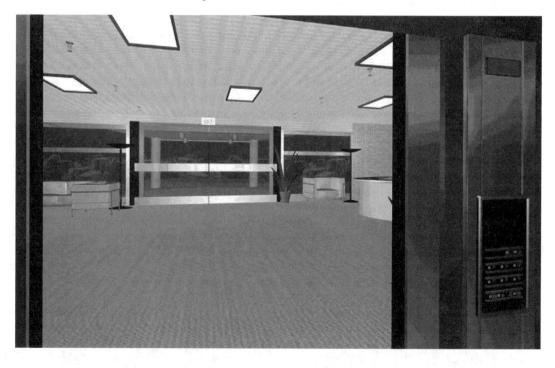

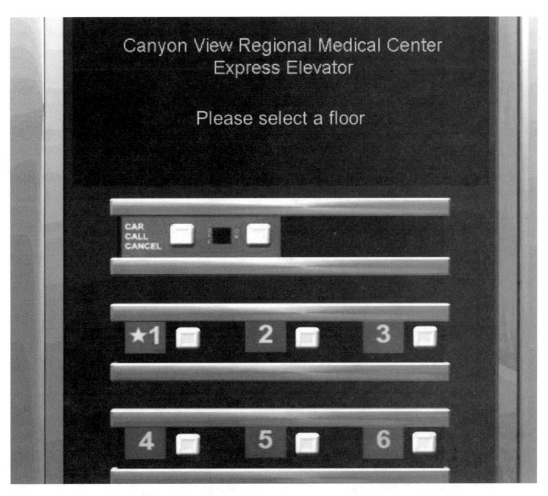

Since you are in a medical-surgical rotation, you will not be able to visit the Well-Child Clinic. However, you can work with two patients on the Pediatric Floor (Disk 1), one patient in the Intensive Care Unit (Disk 2), three patients on the Medical-Surgical/Telemetry Floor (Disk 2), and one who spends time on both the Medical-Surgical/Telemetry Floor and in the Surgery Department (Disk 2).

Now, go to a unit and sign in for patient care. With Disk 2 in your CD-ROM drive, try this:

- Click on the button for the Medical-Surgical/Telemetry Floor, which is Floor 6.
- The elevator takes you to that floor and opens onto a virtual unit with a Nurses' Station in the center and rooms arrayed around the Nurses' Station.
- Click on the **Nurses' Station** and you will be transported behind its counter.
- If you click and hold the mouse button down, you can get a 360° view of the Medical-Surgical/Telemetry floor by dragging your mouse left or right. With the button still held down, drag to the left, then up, then down. You get a complete view of the Nurses' Station and the floor (see p. 8).
- Take a few minutes to familiarize yourself with the Nurses' Station. Find the two computers, one of which has **Login** on its screen. This is the computer that allows you to select a patient. The other computer is the **Electronic Patient Records** terminal. As you look around the Nurses' Station, you also will see the patient Charts, the Kardex plan of care notebooks, and the Medication Administration Record notebook (labeled MAR).

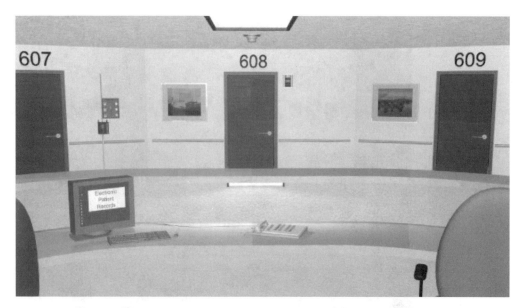

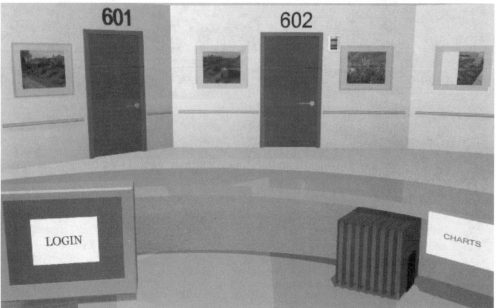

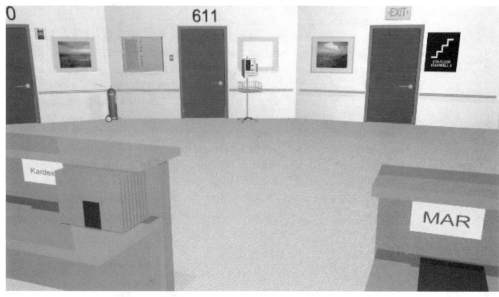

■ WORKING WITH PATIENTS

In *Virtual Clinical Excursions—General Hospital*, the Medical-Surgical/Telemetry floor can be visited between 07:00 and 15:00, but a user can see only one patient at a time and then only in blocks of time. We call these blocks "periods of care." In any of the Medical-Surgical/Telemetry floor scenarios, you can select a patient and a period of care by accessing the Supervisor's (Login) Computer. Double-click on this computer to open the sign-in screen, which contains a box with instructions. Click the **Login** button and you will see a screen that lists the patients on this floor and the periods of care in which you can visit and work with them. Again, only one patient can be selected at a time. When work is completed on that patient, you can select another period of care for that patient or another patient.

Note: During a patient simulation you may receive an on-screen message informing you that the current period of care has ended. If this occurs and you have not yet completed the assigned activities (or if you want to review part of the simulation), you can return to the Supervisor's Computer and sign in again for the same patient and period of care. When the Warning screen appears, click **Erase**. On the other hand, if you simply want to review the data you entered during that period of care, you can sign in for the same patient in a later time period and review data in the EPR. Please note that this option doesn't apply to the final period of care. If you are working with a patient during the last period of care, make sure you keep an eye on the on-screen clock and are aware of how much time is remaining.

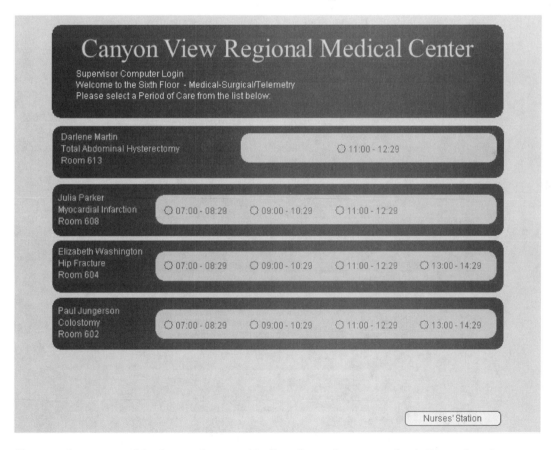

You can choose any of the four patients on this floor (but only one at a time). For each patient you will select a period of care. Three of the patients (Julia Parker, Elizabeth Washington, and Paul Jungerson) can be seen during four periods of care: 07:00–08:29, 09:00–10:29, 11:00–12:29, and 13:00–14:29. You will follow the fourth patient, Darlene Martin, through a Perioperative Rotation. You see her first in the Surgery Department (Floor 4) for a Preoperative Interview (conducted two days prior to surgery). She then goes to the Surgery Department for preoperative care, surgery, and a period in the PACU (09:30–10:29). After leaving PACU, she is transferred to the Medical-Surgical/Telemetry Floor (Floor 6) at 11:00, and you can see her on that floor from 11:00–12:29. There is one patient, James Story, in the Intensive Care Unit (Floor 6).

There are two patients (De Olp and Maria Ortiz) on the Pediatric Floor. Although the patients in the Surgery Department (Floor 4), Intensive Care Unit (Floor 5), and the Medical-Surgical/Telemetry Floor (Floor 6) are all found on Disk 2, the patients on the Pediatric Floor are found on Disk 1. Here are the steps to follow when you need to swap disks:

- If you are currently signed in for a patient, go to the Supervisor's (Login) Computer and sign out. Return to the Nurses' Station.
- Leave the Nurses' Station and enter the elevator. Once you are inside the elevator, remove the disk from your CD-ROM drive and replace it with the other disk.
- Click on the button of the floor number where you need to go.

If you attempt to access the Pediatric Floor (Floor 3) while Disk 2 is in your CD-ROM drive, the computer will eject the disk and prompt you to insert Disk 1 to continue (see below). Likewise, if you attempt to access the Surgery Department, ICU, or the Medical-Surgical/Telemetry Floor while Disk 1 is in your CD-ROM drive, the disk will be ejected and the computer will prompt you to insert Disk 2 to continue.

(*Note:* The process of selecting patients is basically the same on all floors of Canyon View Regional Medical Center, although the available periods of care in the Surgery Department are different from those on the other floors. You will observe this when you visit the other floors.)

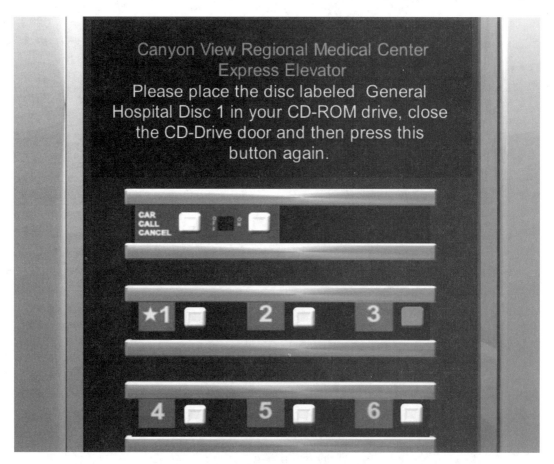

■ PATIENT LIST

◆ Floor 3: Pediatric Floor (Disk 1)

- Maria Ortiz (Room 308)
  Maria is an 8-year-old child who was admitted from the Emergency Department with an acute exacerbation of asthma. She has a 2-year history of asthma. Past acute exacerbation have been treated with Prelone.

- De Olp (Room 310)
  De is a 6-year-old girl who entered the hospital 4 days ago. A bone marrow aspiration confirmed a diagnosis of acute lymphoblastic leukemia. She has had a lumbar puncture for assessment of cerebral spinal fluid, intrathecal chemotherapy, and placement of a Port-a-Cath for administering additional chemotherapy agents.

◆ Floor 4: Surgery Department (Disk 2)

- Darlene Martin
  Ms. Martin is a 49-year-old female who begins Tuesday in the Surgery Department to prepare for a total abdominal hysterectomy. She has been suffering from irregular periods and an enlarged uterus over the past six months, which has caused endometrial hyperplasia. A few days before her surgery, she had a preoperative interview. On Tuesday morning she enters a period of preoperative care, then undergoes a hysterectomy. After a period in the Post-Anesthesia Care Unit (PACU), she is transferred to the Medical-Surgical/Telemetry Floor.

◆ Floor 5: Intensive Care Unit (Disk 2)

- James Story (Room 512)
  Mr. Story is a 42-year-old male who arrived in the Emergency Department complaining of shortness of breath, increasing weakness with a tingling sensation in his extremities, nausea, recent onset of diarrhea, lower leg edema, and a significantly edematous right arm. Mr. Story has type 1 (insulin-dependent) diabetes mellitus and has been undergoing hemodialysis treatment for almost a year. During his stay, he begins experiencing renal failure.

◆ Floor 6: Medical-Surgical/Telemetry Floor (Disk 2)

- Paul Jungerson (Room 602)
  Mr. Jungerson is a 61-year-old male who is recovering from a colon resection. He has a history of diverticulitis, hypertension, pneumonia, and chronic ankle pain.

- Elizabeth Washington (Room 604)
  Ms. Washington is a 63-year-old female who was admitted following an auto accident in which she fractured her hip. She has a history of hypertension and asthma.

- Julia Parker (Room 608)
  Ms. Parker is a 51-year-old female who presented to the Emergency Department with indigestion and mid-back pain. She has a history of hypertension, type 2 diabetes, hyperlipidemia, and obesity. During her stay, she undergoes a heart catheterization and angioplasty, before suffering a myocardial infarction.

- Darlene Martin (Room 613)
  Remember Darlene Martin, the surgical patient? (See Floor 4 above.) After a period in the PACU, Ms. Martin is transferred to the Medical-Surgical/Telemetry Floor.

■ VISITING A PATIENT

Each time you sign in for a new patient and period of care, you enter the simulation at the start of that period of care. The simulations are constructed so that you can conduct a fairly complete assessment of your patient in the first 30 minutes of each period of care. However, after completing a general survey, you should begin to focus your assessments on specific areas. For example, within one period of care you should not do a head-to-toe examination each time you come into a patient's room. Instead, conduct a complete physical at the start of a period of care, then select assessments that are appropriate for your patient's current condition and are based on how that condition is changing. Just as in the real world, a patient's data will change over time as the patient improves or deteriorates. Even if a patient remains stable, there will be diurnal variations in physiology, and these will be reflected in changes in assessment data.

As soon as you sign in to begin working with a patient, a clock appears on screen to help you keep track of time. The clock, which operates in "real time," is located in the bottom left-hand corner of the screen when you are in the Nurses' Station and in the top right-hand corner when you are in the patient's room.

To become familiar with some of the learning resources in *Virtual Clinical Excursions—General Hospital*, insert Disk 2 in your CD-ROM drive, go to Floor 6, select Elizabeth Washington, and choose the 07:00–08:29 period of care. Then click on the button in the lower right corner labeled **Nurses' Station**. This procedure will select the patient and time period for your work. You are then automatically sent to a Case Overview, which provides a short video in which your preceptor introduces the patient. There is also a button labeled **Assignment**. Clicking on this button will open a summary sheet that provides information about the patient and guidance for your work in the simulation.

After completing the Case Overview, you can enter the simulation by clicking on the **Nurses' Station** button in the lower right corner of the screen. This will take you back to the Nurses' Station, where you can begin working with your patient. Remember three things:

- You must select a patient and period of care before any of that patient's simulation and data become available to you.
- Just as in the real world, the Nurses' Station is the base from which you can access patient records and from which you go onto the floor to visit a patient.
- Before you can access another patient simulation, you must go back to the Supervisor's (Login) Computer and follow the procedure to sign out from your current period of care.

Now that you have signed in to care for a patient, Elizabeth Washington, you have several choices. You can enter Elizabeth's room and work with your preceptor to assess the patient. You can review her patient records, which include her Chart, a Kardex plan of care, her active Medication Administration Record (MAR), or the Electronic Patient Record (EPR), all of which contain data that have been collected since Elizabeth entered the hospital. You may know that some hospitals have only paper records and others have only electronic records. Canyon View Regional Medical Center, the virtual hospital, has a combination of paper records (the patient's Chart, Kardex, and MAR) and electronic records (the EPR).

Let's begin by becoming more familiar with the Nurses' Station screen. In the upper left-hand corner, find a menu with these five buttons:

- Patient Care
- Planning Care
- Patient Records
- Case Conference
- Clinical Review

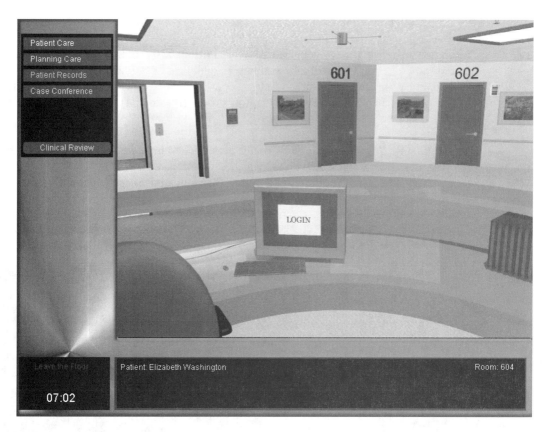

One at a time, single-click on these buttons to reveal drop-down menus with additional options for each item. First, click on **Patient Care**. Two options are available for this item: **Case Overview** and **Data Collection**. You completed the Case Overview after signing in for Ms. Washington, but you can always go back to review it. For example, you might want to return there and click the **Assignment** button to review the summary of Ms. Washington's care up to the start of your shift—or to remind yourself what tasks you have been asked to complete.

◆ **Data Collection**

To conduct an assessment of your patient, click **Patient Care** and then **Data Collection** from the drop-down menu. This will take you into a small anteroom (part of the patient's room) with a sink, laundry bin, and biohazards waste receptacle. *Note:* You can also enter this anteroom by clicking on the outer door of Ms. Washington's room (Room 604). To visit your patient, complete these steps:

- First *wash your hands!* Click on the sink once to indicate you are beginning to wash. Click again to indicate you are finished washing.
- Now click on the curtain to the right of the sink and enter the patient's room.

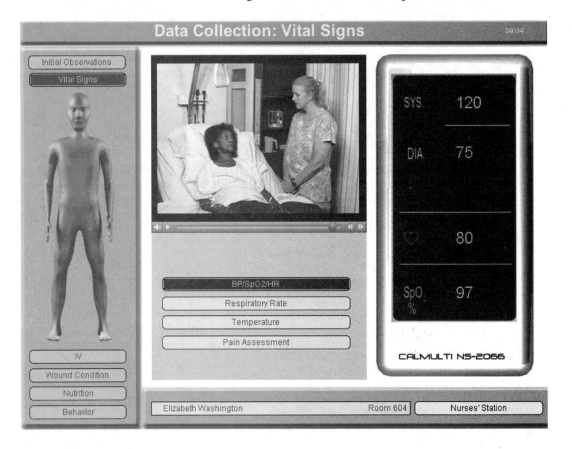

Once in the patient's room, your screen is equipped with various tools you can use for data collection. In the center of the screen, you will see a still frame of your patient. Along the left side of the screen are buttons and a body model that allow you to access learning activities in which your preceptor conducts different types of assessments. Try clicking on the buttons and different body parts. (Note that the body model rotates once your cursor touches it. As you move your cursor over the model, various body parts are highlighted in orange.)

What happened when you clicked on the buttons or body parts? Many of the buttons open options for additional assessments—these always appear below the video screen. Likewise, clicking on a highlighted area of the body model opens options for additional assessments. The body model serves two purposes. First, it provides a way for you to develop a sense of what assessments and physiologic systems are associated with different areas of the human body. Second, it acts as a quick navigational tool that allows you to focus on certain types of assessments.

Note that the body model is a "generic" figure without specific sexual or racial characteristics. However, we encourage you to always think about your patients as unique individuals. The body model is simply a tool designed to help you develop assessment skills by body area and navigate quickly though the simulation's learning activities. Review the diagram below to become familiar with the available Data Collection buttons and the additional options that appear when you click each button and body area.

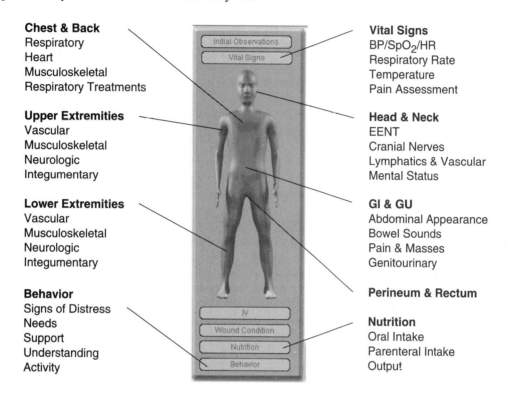

Chest & Back
Respiratory
Heart
Musculoskeletal
Respiratory Treatments

Upper Extremities
Vascular
Musculoskeletal
Neurologic
Integumentary

Lower Extremities
Vascular
Musculoskeletal
Neurologic
Integumentary

Behavior
Signs of Distress
Needs
Support
Understanding
Activity

Vital Signs
BP/SpO₂/HR
Respiratory Rate
Temperature
Pain Assessment

Head & Neck
EENT
Cranial Nerves
Lymphatics & Vascular
Mental Status

GI & GU
Abdominal Appearance
Bowel Sounds
Pain & Masses
Genitourinary

Perineum & Rectum

Nutrition
Oral Intake
Parenteral Intake
Output

Whenever you click on an assessment button, either a video or still photo will be activated in the center of the screen. For some activities, data obtained during assessment are shown in a box to the right of that frame (see p. 14). For other assessment options, you must collect data yourself by observing the video—in these cases, no data appear in the box. You can always replay a video by simply reclicking the assessment button of the activity you wish to see again.

The *Virtual Clinical Excursions—General Hospital* patient simulations were constructed by expert nurses to be as realistic as possible. As previously mentioned, the data for every patient will change through time. During the first 30 minutes of a period of care, you will generally find that all assessment options will give you data on the patient. However, after that period, some assessments may no longer be a high priority for a patient. The expert nurses who created the patient simulations let you know when an assessment area is not a high priority by sending you a short message. These messages appear in the box on the right side of the screen, where data are normally listed. Some examples of messages you might receive include "Please rethink your priorities for assessment of this patient" and "Your assessment should be focused on other areas at this time."

To leave the patient's room, click on the **Nurses' Station** button in the bottom right-hand corner of the screen. Note that this takes you back through the anteroom, where you must wash your hands before leaving. Once you have washed your hands, click on the outer door to return to the Nurses' Station.

Now, let's review what you just learned and try a few quick exercises to get a sense of how the Data Collection learning activities become available to you. You are already signed in to care for Elizabeth Washington, who was admitted following an auto accident in which her hip was fractured. Reenter her room from the Nurses' Station by clicking on **Patient Care** and then on **Data Collection**. You are now in the sink area of the patient's room, so wash your hands and click on the curtain to see the patient.

Start your patient care by collecting Ms. Washington's vital signs.

- Click on **Vital Signs**. Four assessment options will appear below the picture of the patient.
- Click on **BP/SpO$_2$/HR**. Watch the video as your preceptor measures blood pressure, oxygen saturation, and heart rate on a noninvasive multipurpose monitor. Record Ms. Washington's data for these attributes in the chart below.
- Now click on **Respiratory Rate**. This time, after a video plays, a "breathing" body model appears on the right. Measure Ms. Washington's respiratory rate by counting the respirations of the body model for the period of time your instructor recommends. Record your estimate of her respiratory rate below.
- Next, click on **Temperature**. First, you will see your preceptor measuring Ms. Washington's temperature; then the thermometer reading appears in the frame to the right. Record her temperature.
- Finally, assess Ms. Washington's pain by clicking on **Pain Assessment**. Note your interpretation of her pain. If she is in pain, record her pain level and characteristics.

Vital Signs	Time
Blood pressure	
SpO$_2$	
Heart rate	
Respiratory rate	
Temperature	
Pain rating	

Once you have collected Ms. Washington's vital signs, begin a lower extremities examination. Point your cursor to the leg area of the body model. Click anywhere on the orange highlighted area. Four new options now appear below the picture of your patient.

- Click on **Vascular**. Observe the video and review the data you obtain from this examination.
- Now click on **Neurologic**. Is Ms. Washington experiencing any numbness or tingling in her arms or legs?

You have now collected vital signs data and conducted a limited lower extremities assessment of Ms. Washington. As previously mentioned, most of the assessments combine a video or still photo of the patient with data that are collected for the respective assessment. Other assessments simply provide a video, and you must collect data from the nurse-patient interaction. For example, many of the pain assessments consist of the nurse asking the patient to rate his or her pain and the patient responding with a rating. Some of the behavior assessments also require that you listen to the nurse-patient interaction and make a decision about the patient's condition, needs, or psychosocial attributes.

When you visit patients in the Surgery Department, you will notice slightly different assessment options for some periods of care. However, the same types of interactions are always available. When you click on a button or area of the body model, you will be able to access a variety of patient assessments. If a video is shown, it can always be replayed by clicking on the assessment button.

■ HOW TO FIND AND ACCESS A PATIENT'S RECORDS

So far, you have visited a patient and practiced collecting data. Now you will examine the types of available patient records and learn how to access them. The records include the patient Charts, Medication Administration Record (MAR), Kardex plan of care, and Electronic Patient Record (EPR).

You are still signed in for Elizabeth Washington on the Medical-Surgical/Telemetry Floor, so let's explore her records. From the Nurses' Station, each type of patient record can be accessed in two ways. Practice both methods and choose the pathway you prefer. The first option is to use the menu in the upper left corner of the screen. First, click on **Patient Records**; this reveals a drop-down menu. Then select the type of patient record you wish to review by clicking on one of these options:

- **EPR**—Electronic Patient Record
- **Chart**—The patient's chart
- **Kardex**—A Kardex plan of care
- **MAR**—The current Medication Administration Record

You can also access patient records by clicking on various objects in the Nurses' Station. On the counter inside the station you will find a set of charts, a set of Kardex plans of care, a Medication Administration Record notebook, and a computer that houses the Electronic Patient Record system. All objects inside the Nurses' Station are labeled for quick recognition.

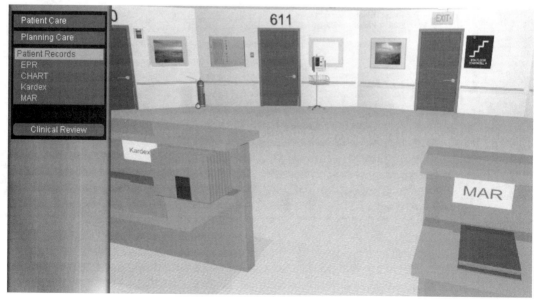

Chart

To open Ms. Washington's chart, click on **Chart** in the **Patient Records** drop-down menu—or click on the stack of Charts inside the Nurses' Station. Colored tabs at the bottom of the screen allow you to navigate through the following sections of the chart:

- History & Physical
- Nursing History
- Admissions Records
- Physician Orders
- Progress Notes
- Laboratory Reports
- X-Rays & Diagnostics
- Operative Reports
- Medication Records
- Consults
- Rehabilitation & Therapy
- Social Services
- Miscellaneous

To flip forward in the chart, select any available tab. Once you have moved beyond the first tab (History & Physical), a **Flip Back** icon appears just above the red cross in the lower right corner. Click on **Flip Back** to return to earlier sections of the chart. The data for each patient's chart are updated during a shift; updates occur at the start of a period of care. Note that some of the records in the chart are several pages long. You will need to scroll down to read all of the pages in some sections of the chart.

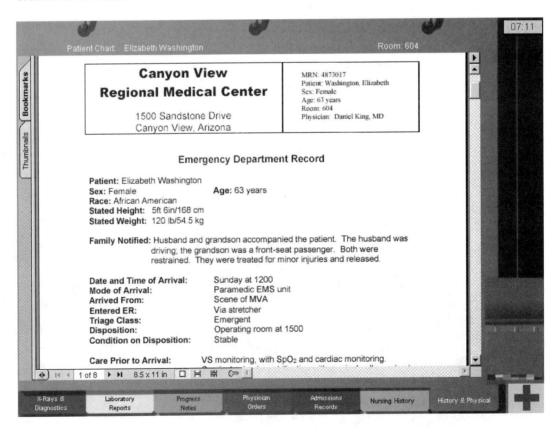

Flipping forward and back through the various sections is accomplished by clicking on the tabs or on the **Flip Back** icon. To close a patient's chart, click on the **Nurses' Station** icon in the lower right corner of the screen.

Medication Administration Record (MAR)

The notebook under the MAR sign in the Nurses' Station contains the active Medication Administration Record for each patient. This record lists the current 24-hour medication orders for each patient. Double-click on the MAR to open it like a notebook. (*Remember:* You can also access the MAR through the Patient Records menu.) Once open, the MAR has tabs that allow you to select patients by room number. Each MAR lists the following information for every medication a patient is receiving:

- Medication name
- Route and dosage of medication
- Time to administer medication

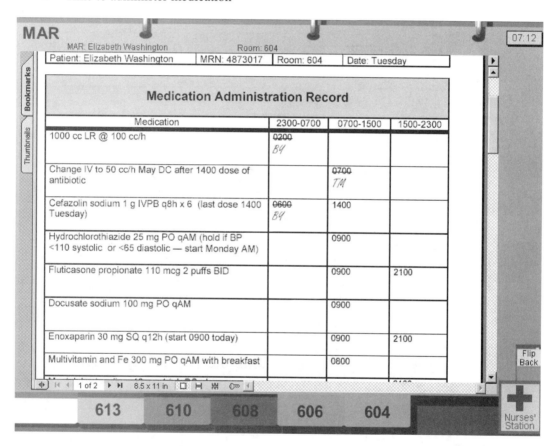

Scroll down to be sure you have read all the data. As with the patient charts, flip forward and back through the MAR by clicking on the patient room tabs or on the **Flip Back** icon. *Note:* Unlike the patient's Chart, which allows you to access data *only* for the patient for whom you are signed in, the MAR allows access to the data for *all* patients on the floor. Because the MAR is arranged numerically by patient room number, it is important that you remember to click on the correct tab for your current patient rather than reading the first record that appears on opening the MAR.

The MAR is updated at the start of every period of care. To close the MAR, click on the **Nurses' Station** icon in the lower right corner of the screen.

Kardex Plan of Care

Most hospitals keep a notebook in the Nurses' Station with each patient's plan of care. Canyon View Regional Medical Center's simplified plan of care is a three-page document modeled after the Kardex forms often used in hospitals. Access the Kardex through the drop-down menu (click **Patient Records**, then **Kardex**), or click on the folders beneath the Kardex sign in the Nurses' Station. *Note:* Like the MAR, the Kardex allows access to the plans of care for *all* patients on the floor. Side tabs allow you to select the patient's care plan by room number. Remember to click on the tab for your current patient rather than reading the first plan of care that appears after opening the Kardex. Scroll down to read all of the pages.

A Flip Back icon appears in the upper right corner once you have moved past the first patient's Kardex. Use the Nurses' Station icon in the bottom right corner to return to close the Kardex.

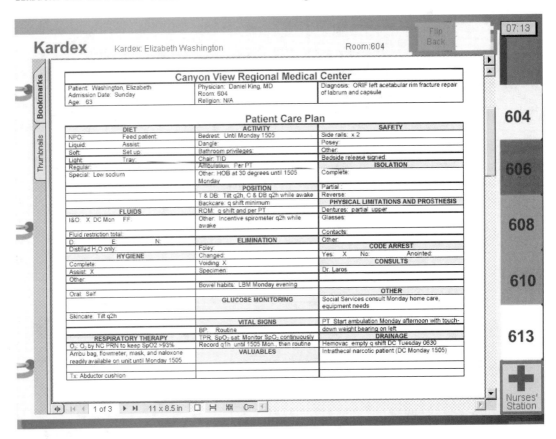

Electronic Patient Record (EPR)

Some patient records are kept in a computerized system called the Electronic Patient Record (EPR). Although some hospitals have only limited electronic patient records—or none at all— most hospitals are moving toward computerized or electronic patient record systems.

The Canyon View EPR was designed to represent a composite of commercial versions used in existing hospitals and clinics. If you have already used an EPR in a hospital, you will recognize the basic features of all commercial or custom-designed EPRs. If you have not used an EPR, the Canyon View system will give you an introduction to a basic computerized record system.

You can use the EPR to review data already recorded for a patient—or to enter assessment data that you have collected. The EPR is continually updated. For example, when you begin working with a patient for the 11:00–12:29 period of care, you have access to all the data for that patient up to 11:00. The EPR contains all data collected on the patient from the moment he or she entered the hospital. The Canyon View EPR allows you to examine how data for different attributes have changed during the time the patient has been in the hospital. You may also examine data for all of a patient's attributes at a particular time. Remember, the Canyon View EPR is fully functional, as in a real hospital. Just as in real life, you can enter data during the period of care in which you are working, but you cannot change data from a previous period of care.

You can access the EPR once you have signed in for a patient. Use the Patient Records menu or find the computer in the Nurses' Station with **Electronic Patient Records** on the screen. To access a patient's EPR:

- Select the EPR option on the drop-down menu (click **Patient Records**, then **EPR**) or double-click on the EPR computer screen. This will open the access screen.
- Type in the password—this will always be **nurse2b**—but *Do Not Hit Return* after entering the password.
- Click on the **Access Records** button.
- If you make a mistake, simply delete the password, reenter it, and click **Access Records**.

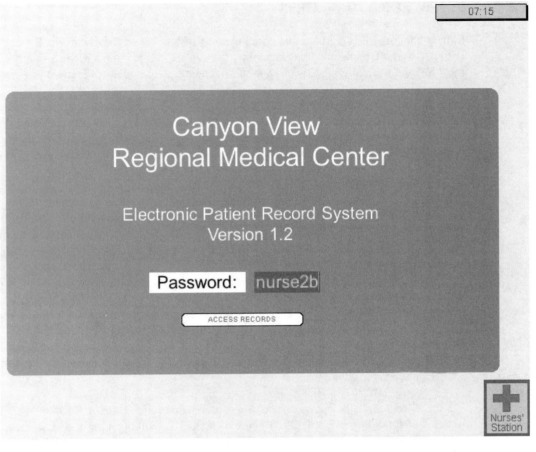

At the bottom of the EPR screen, you will see buttons for various types of patient data. Clicking on a button will bring up a field of attributes and the data for those attributes. You may notice that the data for some attributes appear as codes. The appropriate codes (and interpretations) for any attributes can be found in the code box on the far right side of the screen. Remember that every hospital or clinic selects its own codes. The codes used by Canyon View Regional Medical Center may be different from ones you have used or seen in clinical rotations. However, you will have to adjust to the various codes used by the clinical settings in which you work, so *Virtual Clinical Excursions—General Hospital* gives you some practice using a system different from one you may already know. The different data fields available in the EPR are:

- Vital Signs
- Neurologic
- Musculoskeletal
- Respiratory
- Cardiovascular
- GI & GU
- IV
- Equipment
- Drains & Tubes
- Wounds & Dressings
- Hygiene
- Safety & Comfort
- Behavior & Activity
- Intake & Output

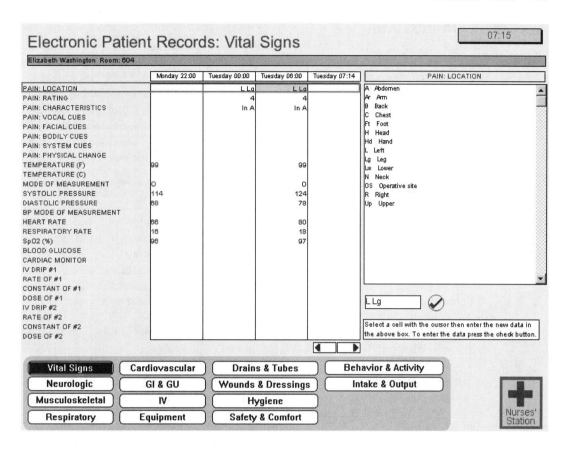

Click on **Vital Signs** and review the vital signs data for Elizabeth Washington. If you want to enter data you have collected for a particular attribute (such as pain characteristics), click on the data field in which the attribute is found. (Pain characteristics are found in the Vital Signs field.) Then click on the specific attribute line, and move the highlighted box to the current time cell. Blue arrows in the lower right corner move you left and right within the EPR data fields. Once the highlighted box is in the correct time cell, type in the code for your patient's pain characteristics in the box at the lower right side of the screen, just to the left of the check mark (√). Be sure to use the codes listed in the code box in the data entry area. Once you have typed the data in this box, click on the check mark (√) to enter and save them in the patient's record. The data will appear in the time cell for the attribute you have selected.

When you are ready to leave the EPR, click on the **Nurses' Station** icon in the bottom right corner of the screen.

■ PLANNING CARE

After assessing your patient, you must begin the careful process of deciding what diagnoses best describe his or her condition. For each diagnosis, you will list outcomes that you want your patient to achieve. Then, based on each outcome, you will select nursing interventions that you believe will help your patient achieve the outcomes you selected. *Virtual Clinical Excursions—General Hospital* helps you in this process by providing a set of Planning Care resources. While you are still signed in for Elizabeth Washington, click on **Planning Care** in the upper left corner of the Nurses' Station screen. You will see two options: **Problem Identification** and **Setting Priorities**.

◆ Developing Nursing Diagnoses

Click on **Problem Identification**, and a note from your preceptor appears offering guidance about Ms. Washington's problems and possible diagnoses for the types of problems she may have. This diagnosis list is based on what expert nurses believe are *possible* for this particular patient. Remember, however, that not all of the diagnoses listed may apply to your patient—and that your patient may have other diagnoses that are not on the list. Your challenge and responsibility is to decide what nursing diagnoses *do* apply to your patient during each period of care. Since your patient's condition may be changing, some diagnoses may apply in one period of care but not in another. Read over the list of possible diagnoses for Elizabeth Washington. When you are finished, click on **Nurses' Station** to close the Problem Identification note.

Click again on **Planning Care**. This time select **Setting Priorities**. This will open another note from your preceptor. Notice that in the third paragraph of the note, your preceptor instructs you to use the Nursing Care Matrix. This is a resource designed to help you develop nursing diagnoses for your patient. To see how this resource works, click on the **Nursing Care Matrix** button at the bottom of the screen. Before you can develop nursing diagnoses, you must be sure your patient actually has the characteristics of those diagnoses. It is nearly impossible for anyone to remember all of the defining characteristics for every diagnosis, so nurses consult references such as *Nursing Diagnoses: Definitions and Classification, 2001–2002* (NANDA, 2001). To make your life a little simpler and to provide training in the health informatics resources of the future, the Nursing Care Matrix provides a list of diagnoses common for your type of patient, as well as the definition for each diagnosis and the defining characteristics for each diagnosis. Ackley and Ladwig (*Nursing Diagnosis Handbook: A Guide to Planning Care*, 5th edition) have mapped specific NANDA diagnoses onto major health-illness transitions. This mapping, along with input from our expert panel of nurses, provided the list of diagnoses you see—nursing diagnoses that *might* apply to Elizabeth Washington.

- Click on the first diagnosis. Note that the definition for this diagnosis now appears in a box in the upper right of the screen. The defining characteristics are listed in the box in the lower right of the screen.
- Click on another diagnosis. Review the definition and characteristics.

◆ Developing Outcomes and Interventions

For every nursing diagnosis you make, you can then select appropriate outcomes that you want your patient to achieve.

- Click on a diagnosis.
- Now click on **Outcomes and Interventions** at the bottom of the screen.
- On the left-hand side of the screen, you should now see the diagnosis you selected, along with a list of the outcomes you may want your patient to achieve if she has this diagnosis.

These outcomes are based on *Nursing Outcomes Classification*, 2nd edition (Johnson, Maas, and Moorhead, 2000). This reference provides detailed lists of linkages between the NANDA diagnoses and nursing outcomes defined in the *Nursing Outcomes Classification*.

For each outcome listed, you can access a list of nursing interventions to help your patient achieve that outcome.

- Click on the first outcome listed.
- On the right side of your screen, you will now see lists of intervention labels in three boxes: Major Interventions, Suggested Interventions, and Optional Interventions.

Each of the intervention labels in these boxes refers to an intervention that could be implemented to help achieve the specific outcome chosen. The *Nursing Intervention Classification* system gives a label to each intervention. Therefore, the Major, Suggested, and Optional Interventions are labels, each of which has a set of nursing activities that together comprise an intervention. If you look up a label in the *Nursing Interventions Classification*, you will see that it refers to a set of different nursing activities, some or all of which can be implemented in order to achieve the desired patient outcome for that diagnosis. We used *Nursing Diagnoses, Outcomes, and Interventions: NANDA, NOC and NIC Linkages* (Johnson, Bulechek, McCloskey-Dochterman, Mass, and Moorhead, 2001) and the *Nursing Interventions Classification*, 3rd edition, (McCloskey and Bulechek, 2000) to create the linkages between outcomes and interventions shown in the Nursing Care Matrix.

The Nursing Care Matrix provides you with a basic framework for learning how to move from making a diagnosis to defining patient outcomes and then to choosing the interventions you should implement to achieve those outcomes. Your instructor and the exercises in this workbook will help you develop this part of the nursing process and will provide you with more information about the nursing activities that belong with each intervention label.

■ CLINICAL REVIEW

Virtual Clinical Excursions—General Hospital also incorporates a learning assessment system called the Clinical Review, which provides quizzes that evaluate your knowledge of your patient's condition and related conditions.

- If you are still in the Nursing Care Matrix, return to the Nurses' Station by clicking first on **Return to Diagnoses** at the bottom of the Outcomes and Interventions screen and then on **Return to Nurses' Station** at the bottom of the Diagnosis screen.
- From the menu options in the upper left corner, click on **Clinical Review**.
- You will now see a warning box that asks you to confirm that you wish to continue. Click **Clinical Review Center**.

You are now looking at the opening screen for the Clinical Review Center. You have three quiz options: **Safe Practice**, **Nursing Diagnoses**, and **Clinical Judgment**. Do not click on any quiz buttons yet. First, read the following descriptions of the quizzes you can select:

- **Safe Practice**
  The **Safe Practice** quiz presents you with NCLEX-type questions based on the patient you worked with during this period of care. A set of five questions is randomly drawn from a pool of questions. Answer the questions, and the Clinical Review Center will score your performance.

- **Nursing Diagnoses**
  If you click on the **Nursing Diagnoses** button, you are presented with a list of 20 NANDA nursing diagnoses. You must select the five diagnoses in this list that most likely apply to your patient. The Clinical Review Center records your choices, gathers those choices that are correct, and scores your performance. The quiz then allows you to select nursing interventions for each of the outcomes associated with NANDA diagnoses that your correctly chose. For each of your correct diagnoses, you are presented with the likely outcomes for that diagnosis; for each outcome, you will see a list of six

nursing intervention labels. Only three of the intervention labels are appropriate for each outcome. You must select the correct labels. Again, your performance is automatically scored.

- **Clinical Judgment**
  The **Clinical Judgment** quiz asks you to consider a single question. This question evaluates your understanding of your patient's condition during the period of care in which you have just worked. Select your answer from four options related to your perception of your patient's stability and the frequency of monitoring you should be conducting.

You can take one, two, or all three of the quizzes. On any floor, when you are done with the quizzes, you must click on **Finish**. This will take you to a **Preceptor's Evaluation**, which offers a scorecard of your performance on the quizzes, discusses your understanding of the patient's condition and related conditions, and makes recommendations for you to improve your understanding.

Preceptor's Evaluation

	Clinical Review	
	Correct Responses	Score
Safe Practice	3.0	18.0
Implementing Nursing Care	4.0	16.0
Clinical Judgment	1.0	20.0
Totals		54.0
Total Score	Out of 100 possible points, you received 54.0 points or 54.0%	

Preceptor's Evaluation of Clinical Review

Clincial Judgment Recommendation - Congratulations! You made a good clinical decision about your client during this period of care

We want you to spend time practicing questions like those found in the Safe Practice assessment. These questions are very similar to those found on the NCLEX-RN. Also, we feel you need to study the nursing diagnoses approved by the North American Nursing Diagnosis Association (NANDA). Importantly, we want you to review the outcomes appropriate for a particular diagnosis as well as the interventions you would implement to achieve each outcome. You might want to spend time re-examining the diagnoses-outcomes-interventions linkages found in the Nursing Care Matrix. As mentioned above, the nursing diagnoses are based on approved diagnoses of the North American Nursing Diagnosis Association (NANDA). Remember that the outcomes are based on the Nursing Outcomes Classification and the interventions are based on the Nursing Interventions Classification (NIC).

Print a detailed report   Nurses' Station

Note: We don't recommend that you take any quizzes before working with a patient. The goal of *Virtual Clinical Excursions—General Hospital* is to help you learn and prepare for practice as a professional nurse. Reading your textbook, using this workbook to complete the CD-ROM activities, and organizing your thoughts about your patient's condition will help you prepare for the quizzes. More important, this work will help you prepare for care of real-life patients in clinical settings.

■ HOW TO QUIT OR CHANGE PATIENTS

Eventually, you will want to take a short or long break, begin caring for a different patient, or exit the software.

◆ To Take a Short Break

- Go to the Nurses' Station.
- Click on **Leave the Floor**, an icon in the lower left corner of the screen.
- You will see a screen with a variety of options.
- Click on **Break** and you will be given a 10-minute break. This stops the clock. After 10 minutes you are automatically returned to the floor, where you reenter the simulation at the same moment in time that you left.

◆ To Change Patients

Choose option 1 or option 2 below, depending on which activities you have completed during this period of care.

1. Use the following instructions *if you have already completed one or more of the quizzes* in the Clinical Review Center for your current patient:

   - Double-click on the **Supervisor's (Login) Computer** in the Nurses' Station.
   - Read the instructions for logging in for a new patient and period of care.
   - If you want to select a new patient on the *same* floor, click **Login**, select the new patient and period of care, and then click **Nurses' Station**.
   - If you want to work with a patient on a *different* floor, click **Return to Nurses' Station**, take the elevator to the new floor, and sign in for the new patient on the Login computer in the Nurses' Station.

2. Use the following instructions *if you have* not *completed any of the quizzes* in the Clinical Review Center for your current patient:

   - Double-click on the **Supervisor's (Login) Computer** in the Nurses' Station.
   - Read the instructions in the Warning box. Then click on **Supervisor's Computer**.
   - The computer logs you off and gives you the option of going to the Clinical Review Center or to the Nurses' Station. Unless you wish to go to the Clinical Review Center for evaluation of the period of care you just completed, click on **Nurses' Station**.
   - Double-click on the **Login Computer** again, and follow the instructions to sign in for another patient. (See the third and fourth bullets in option 1 above for specific steps.)

When you visit the patients on the Pediatric Floor (Floor 3), you will need to swap disks by following these steps:

- If up are currently signed in for a patient, go to the Supervisor's (Login) Computer and sign out. Return to the Nurses' Station.

- Leave the Nurses' Station and enter the elevator. Once you are inside the elevator, remove the disk from your CD-ROM drive and replace it with the other disk.

- Click on the button of the floor number where you need to go.

◆ **To Quit the Software for a Long Break or to Reset a Simulation**

- From the Nurses' Station, click on **Leave the Floor** in the lower left corner of the screen.
- You will see a new screen with a variety of options.
- You may select Quit with Bookmark or Quit with Reset.
  - **Quit with Bookmark** allows you to leave the simulation and return at the same virtual time you left. Any data you entered in the EPR will remain intact. Choose this option if you want to stop working for more than 10 minutes but wish to reenter the floor later at the exact point at which you left.
  - **Quit with Reset** allows you to quit and reset the simulation. This option erases any data you entered in the EPR during your current session. Choose this option if you know you will be starting a new simulation when you return.

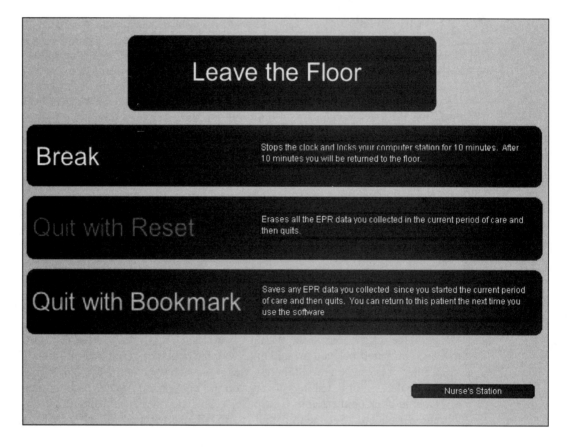

◆ **To Practice Exiting the Software**

- Click **Leave the Floor**.
- Now click **Quit with Reset**.
- A small message box will appear to confirm that you wish to quit and erase any data collected or recorded.
  - If you have reached this message in error, click the red X in the upper right corner to close this box. You may now choose one of the other options for leaving the floor (Break or Quit with Bookmark).
  - If you *do* wish to Quit with Reset, click **OK** on the message box.
- *Virtual Clinical Excursions—General Hospital* will close, and you will be returned to your computer's desktop screen.

A DETAILED TOUR

What do you experience when you care for patients during a clinical rotation? Well, you may be assigned one or several patients that need your attention. You follow the nursing process, assessing your patients, diagnosing each patient's problems or areas of concern, planning their care and setting outcomes you hope they will achieve, implementing care based on the outcomes you have set, and then evaluating the outcomes of your care. It is important to remember that the nursing process is not a static, one-time series of steps. Instead, you loop through the process again and again, continually assessing your patient, reaffirming your earlier diagnoses and perhaps finding improvement in some areas and new problems in other areas, adjusting your plan of care, implementing care as planned or implementing a revised plan, and evaluating patient outcomes to decide whether your patients are achieving expected outcomes. Patient care is hands-on, action-packed, often complex, and sometimes frightening. You must be prepared and present—physically, intellectually, and emotionally.

Textbooks help you build a foundation of knowledge about patient care. Clinical rotations help you apply and extend that book-based learning to the real world. You will know this with certainty when you experience it yourself—for example, when you first read about starting an IV but then have to start an IV on an actual patient, or when you read about the adverse effects of a medication and you then observe these adverse effects emerging in a patient. Stepping from a book onto a hospital floor seems difficult and unsettling. *Virtual Clinical Excursions—General Hospital* is designed as an intermediate tool to help you make the transition from book-based learning to the real world of patient care. The CD-ROM activities provide you with the practice necessary to make that transition by letting you apply your book-based knowledge to virtual patients in simulated settings and situations. Each simulation was developed by an expert nurse or nurse-physician team and is based on realistic patient problems, with a rich variety of data that can be collected during assessment of the patient.

Several types of patient records are available for you to access and analyze. This workbook, the software, and your textbook work together to allow you to move from ***book-based learning*** to real-life ***problem-based learning***. Your foundational knowledge is based on what you have learned from the textbook. The *VCE—General Hospital* patient simulations allow you to explore this knowledge in the context of a virtual hospital with virtual patients. Questions stimulated by the software can be answered by consulting your textbook or reviewing a patient simulation. The workbook is similar to a map or guide, providing a means of connecting textbook content to the practice of skills, data collection, and data interpretation by leading you through a variety of relevant activities based on simulated patients' conditions.

To better understand how *Virtual Clinical Excursions—General Hospital* can help you in your transition, take the following detailed tour, in which you visit three different patients.

■ WORKING WITH A MEDICAL-SURGICAL FLOOR PATIENT

In *Virtual Clinical Excursions—General Hospital*, the Pediatric Floor, the Intensive Care Unit, and Medical-Surgical/Telemetry Floor can be visited between 07:00 and 15:00, but you can care for only one patient at a time and only in the following blocks of time, which we call *periods of care*: 07:00–08:29, 09:00–10:29, 11:00–12:29, and 13:00–14:29. For each clinical simulation, you will select a single patient and a period of care. When you have completed the assigned care for that patient, you can then select a new patient and period of care. You can also reset a simulation at any point and work through the same period of care as many times as you want. Each time you sign in for a patient and time period, you will enter that session at the beginning of that period of care (unless you have previously "saved" a session by choosing Break or Quit with Bookmark).

Consider, for a moment, a typical Intesive Care Unit during the period between 07:00 and 15:00. Suppose that you could accompany a preceptor on that floor and provide care for patients during that 8-hour shift. Different expert nurses might take slightly different approaches, but almost certainly each nurse would establish priorities for patient care. These priorities would be based on report during shift change, a review of the patient records, and the nurse's own assessment of each patient.

At the beginning of a period of care, the assessment of each patient is usually accomplished by a general survey, that is, a fairly complete assessment of a patient's physical and psychosocial status. After the general survey, a nurse subsequently conducts focused assessments during the rest of the shift. The specific types of data collected in such focused assessments are determined by the nurse's interpretation of each patient's condition, needs, and applicable clinical pathways for independent and collaborative care. Depending on an agency's protocols and standards of care for the ICU patient, a nurse may conduct more than one comprehensive assessment during a shift, with focused surveys completed between the general surveys. Regardless of individual agency protocol, any ICU patient would have at least one general survey and numerous focused surveys over the period of the shift.

Now let's put these guidelines to practice by entering the ICU (Disk 2) at Canyon View Regional Medical Center. This time, you will care for James Story, a 42-year-old male suffering from renal failure.

1. Enter and Sign In for James Story

- Insert your *VCE—General Hospital* Disk 2 in your CD-ROM drive and double-click on the **VCE—General Hospital** icon on your desktop. Wait for the program to load.
- When Canyon View Regional Medical Center appears on your screen, click on the hospital entrance to enter the lobby.
- Click on the elevator. Once inside, click on the panel to the right of the door; then click on button **5** for the Intensive Care Unit (ICU).
- When the elevator opens onto the Intensive Care Unit, click on the **Nurses' Station**.
- Inside the Nurses' Station, double-click on the **Supervisor's (Login) Computer** and select James Story as your patient for the 09:00–10:29 period of care.

2. Case Overview

- Signing in automatically takes you to the patient's Case Overview. Your preceptor will appear and speak briefly on the video screen.
- Listen to the preceptor; then click on **Assignment** below the video screen.
- You will now see a Preceptor Note, which is a summary of care for James Story, covering the period of care just before the one you are now working.
- Review the summary of care. Scroll down to read the entire report.
- On the next page, make note of any information that you feel is important or that will require follow-up work, either with the patient or through examination of his records.

Areas of Concern for James Story:

- When you have finished the case overview, click on **Nurses' Station** in the lower right corner of the screen and you will find yourself in the ICU Nurses' Station.

3. Initial Impressions

Visit your patient immediately to get an initial impression of his condition.

- On the menu in the upper left corner of your screen, click on **Patient Care**. From the options on the drop-down menu, click on **Data Collection**. *Remember:* You can also visit the patient by double-clicking on the door to his room (Room 512).
- In the anteroom, wash your hands by double-clicking on the sink. Then click on the curtain to enter the patient area.
- Inside the room, you will see many different options for assessing this patient. First, click on **Initial Observations** in the top left corner of the screen. Observe and listen to the interaction between the nurse preceptor and the patient. Note any areas of concern, issues, or assessments that you may want to pursue later.
- Now that you have gotten an initial impression of your patient, you have a few choices. In some cases, you might wish to leave the patient and access his records to develop a better understanding of his condition and what has happened since he was admitted. However, let's stay with Mr. Story a while longer to conduct a few physical and psychosocial assessments.

4. Vital Signs

Obtain a full set of vital signs from James Story.

- Click on **Vital Signs** (just below the Initial Observations button). This activates a pathway that allows you to measure all or just some of your patient's vital signs. Four options now appear under the picture of James Story. Clicking on any of these options will begin a data collection sequence (usually a short video) in which the respective vital sign is measured. The vital signs data change over time to reflect the temporal changes you would find in a patient such as Mr. Story. Try the various vital signs options to see what kinds of data are obtained.
  - First, click on **BP/SpO$_2$/HR**. Wait for the video to begin; then observe as the nurse preceptor uses a noninvasive monitor to measure Mr. Story's blood pressure, SpO$_2$, and heart rate. After the video stops, the preceptor's findings appear as digital readings on a monitor to the right of the video screen. Record these data in the chart below. If you want to replay the video, simply click again on **BP/SpO$_2$/HR**. *Note:* You can replay any video in this manner—as often as needed.
  - Now click on **Respiratory Rate**. This time, after the video plays, an image of a breathing body model appears on the right. Count the respirations for the amount of time recommended by your instructor. Record your measurement below.
  - Next, click on **Temperature**. Again, a video shows the nurse preceptor obtaining this vital sign, and the result is shown on a close-up of a digital thermometer on the right side of the screen. Record this finding in the chart below.
  - Finally, click on **Pain Assessment** and observe as the nurse preceptor asks Mr. Story about his pain. Note Mr. Story's response in the chart below.

Vital Signs	Time
Blood pressure	
SpO$_2$	
Heart rate	
Respiratory rate	
Temperature	
Pain rating	

5. Mental Status

From some of your vital signs assessments, you should be starting to form an idea of Mr. Story's mental status. However, you can check his mental status more specifically by doing the following:

- On the left side of the Data Collection screen is a body model. When you move your cursor along the body, it begins to rotate and the area beneath your cursor is highlighted in orange.
- Place your cursor on the head area of the body model and click.
- Notice that new assessment options now appear under the picture of your patient.
- Click on **Mental Status** (the bottom option of the list).
- Observe Mr. Story's responses and interactions with the nurse. Then review the data, if any, that appear to the right after the video has stopped.

6. Respiratory Assessment

Auscultate Mr. Story's lungs to see whether there is any evidence of adventitious lung sounds.

- Click on the chest area of the body model.
- Note the new assessment options that come up beneath the picture of Mr. Story.
- Click on **Respiratory**.
- Observe the examination of the anterior, lateral, and posterior chest. Then review the data collected by your preceptor.
- Do you believe there is any evidence of problems? If so, explain what data support your conclusion.
- If you were worried about potential problems, what other assessments might you conduct?

7. Behavior

Since this is your first visit with Mr. Story, you may also want to collect some psychosocial data.

- At the bottom left corner of the screen, click on **Behavior**.
- One at a time, click on each of the behavioral assessment options that appear below the picture of Mr. Story.
- As you observe each assessment, take notes on the nurse-patient interactions.
- Do any of his responses concern you?
- Does he have family support as well as nursing support?
- What other questions do you want to ask Mr. Story? When might you ask these questions?

8. Chart

You have conducted your preliminary examination of James Story. Next, review his patient records.

- To access the patient Charts, either click on the stack of charts inside the Nurses' Station or click on **Patient Records** and then **Chart** from the drop-down menu.
- James Story's Chart automatically appears since you are signed in to care for him. As described earlier in **A Quick Tour**, the Chart is divided into several sections. Each section is marked by a colored tab at the bottom of the screen. To flip forward and back through the Chart sections, click on the labeled tabs and on the **Flip Back** icon, respectively. Once you have moved beyond a section, the tab for that section disappears. You can move back to previous sections *only* by clicking on the **Flip Back** icon, which appears above the Nurses' Station icon in the lower right corner.

- Review the following sections of Mr. Story's chart: History & Physical, Nursing History, Operative Reports, and Progress Notes.
- Based on your analyses of these records and your preliminary assessment of Mr. Story, summarize key issues for this patient's care in the box below.
- When you are finished, close the chart by clicking on the **Nurses' Station** icon.

Key Issues for Patient Care:

---

9. Electronic Patient Record (EPR)

Now examine the data in James Story's EPR.

- To access the EPR, first click **Patient Records** in the upper left corner of the screen. Then click **EPR** on the drop-down menu. *Remember:* As an alternative, you can also double-click on the EPR computer in the Nurses' Station. This computer is located to the left of the Kardex and has **Electronic Patient Records** on the screen.
- On the EPR access screen, enter the password—**nurse2b**—and click **Access Records**.
- The EPR automatically opens to the patient's Vital Signs summary. Examine James Story's vital signs data for the past 8 hours.
- Now click **Respiratory** (three buttons below Vital Signs). The data from assessments of Mr. Story's respiratory system are now shown.
- Examine Mr. Story's data. Record your findings in the box on the next page.

Lung Sounds During the Past 24 Hours:

- Next, click on **Cardiovascular**.
- Review data collected for edema.
- List any evidence for fluid retention as evidenced by edema.
- If edema was observed, make sure you note the location(s) and quality.
- Note any other data that indicate problems.
- Now, make an assessment of Mr. Story's clinical status:

Cardiovascular Data:

---

a. Are any of the vital signs data you collected this morning significantly different from the baselines for those vital signs?

   Circle One: Yes   No

b. If "Yes," which data are different?

c. Do you have any concerns about the data collected during your respiratory assessment?

   Circle One: Yes   No

d. If you answered "No," what data tell you the patient is stable?

e. If you answered "Yes," what are your concerns?

10. Medication Administration Record (MAR)

- James Story has been taking a number of medications. Access his current MAR by double-clicking on the notebook below the MAR sign in the Nurse' Station. You can also open the MAR by clicking on **Patient Records** and then on **MAR** on the drop-down menu.
- Once the MAR notebook is open, access Mr. Story's records by clicking on the tab with his room number (512) at the bottom of the screen.
- Examine the MAR and note any medications that Mr. Story should be given during the period of care between 09:00 and 10:29. Make a list of these medications, the times they are to be administered, and any assessments you should conduct before and after giving the medications.

> Medication Data:
>
>
>
>
>
>
>
>
>

- Click the **Nurses' Station** icon to close the MAR.

11. Planning Care

So far, you have completed a preliminary examination of James Story and reviewed some of his records. Now you can begin to plan his care. *Note:* Before *actually* starting a plan of care, you would conduct a more thorough assessment and a more complete review of this patient's records. However, let's continue so that you can learn how to use *Virtual Clinical Excursion's* unique and valuable Planning Care resource.

- On the drop-down menu, click **Planning Care** and then **Problem Identification**.
- Read the Preceptor Note for James Story and write one nursing diagnosis that you think might apply to this patient. Base your decision on your preliminary assessment and review of his records.

> Nursing Diagnosis:
>
>
>
>

- Click on **Nurses' Station** to close this note.
- Click again on **Planning Care** in the upper left corner of your screen. This time, select **Setting Priorities** from the drop-down menu.
- Review the Preceptor Note on setting priorities for James Story.
- When you have finished, click on **Nursing Care Matrix** at the bottom of your screen.
- You will now see a list of nursing diagnoses approved by the North American Nursing Diagnosis Association (NANDA) that may apply to Mr. Story's condition.
- Find the diagnosis you just identified for Mr. Story. Click on this diagnosis.

- Review the nursing diagnosis definition and the defining characteristics that now appear on the right side of the screen.
- Does the definition fit your patient?
- Does your patient have the defining characteristics? If not, perhaps your assessment was not complete enough for you to make this decision. What other assessments should you conduct in order to determine whether this diagnosis applies to James Story?
- For now, assume that your diagnosis *does* apply to Mr. Story. Click on the **Outcomes and Interventions** button at the bottom of the screen.
- You now see a screen that lists nursing outcomes for your diagnosis. These are based on the Nursing Outcomes Classification. If your patient has this diagnosis, these are the outcomes you will want him to achieve.
- Some or all of these outcomes will probably apply to your patient if he does indeed have the nursing diagnosis you selected.
- Click on the first outcome, and text will appear in the three boxes on the right side of the screen. These boxes show the Major, Suggested, and Optional Interventions that could be implemented to achieve the outcome you selected, based on the Nursing Interventions Classification. *Remember:* Each entry listed in these boxes is an intervention label that represents a *set* of nursing activities that you would implement.
- Review the nursing interventions, especially those in the Major Interventions box. These are the most likely interventions you would implement to achieve the outcome you have clicked. However, you should consider all of the interventions before deciding which apply to the outcome for your patient.
- Now click on **Return to Diagnoses**. At this time, you can explore other diagnoses and their respective outcomes and interventions, or you can click **Return to Nurses' Station**.

Your work with James Story is completed for now. To quit the software and reset a simulation:

- Go to the Nurses' Station.
- Click on **Leave the Floor** in the lower left corner of the screen.
- A screen appears with a variety of options.
- Select **Quit with Reset**, which allows you to quit and reset the simulation. This option erases any data you entered in the EPR during your current session.

■ WORKING WITH A PERIOPERATIVE PATIENT

One of the patients at Canyon View Regional Medical Center, Darlene Martin, has been admitted to undergo a total abdominal hysterectomy.

- In the Surgery Department (Disk 2) on Floor 4, sign in to visit Darlene Martin for her Preoperative Interview.
- After viewing the Case Overview and reading the Assignment, return to the Nurses' Station. Click on **Patient Care** and then **Data Collection** on the drop-down menu.
- Wash your hands, enter the room, and click **View Interview**.
- After observing the interview, click on **Summary** and read the Preceptor Note.
- Now return to the Nurses' Station and sign out of this period of care.
- Click on the **Supervisor's (Login) Computer** again and sign in to visit Ms. Martin during her preoperative care.
- Although you cannot observe Ms. Martin's surgery, you can see her now in the Preoperative Care Bay and later in the PACU
- Once Ms. Martin is transferred out of PACU, you can visit her in her room on the Medical-Surgical/Telemetry Floor (Floor 6).

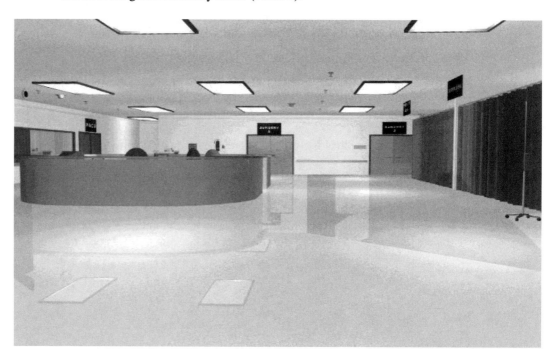

- Spend some time in each of the different perioperative settings in the Surgery Department, as described on p. 38. Then compare these perioperative settings with the settings on the Pediatric Floor and the Medical-Surgical/Telemetry Floor. Use the following chart and focus your comparisons on the themes listed in the left column.

Comparison of Settings in Canyon View Regional Medical Center			
Activities and Resources	Perioperative Settings	Pediatric Floor Settings	Medical-Surgical/ Telemetry Floor Settings
Patient Assessments			
Planning Care			
Types of Patient Records			

Remember: *Virtual Clinical Excursions—General Hospital* is designed to provide a realistic learning environment. Within Canyon View Regional Medical Center, you will not necessarily find the same type of patient records, clinical settings, Nurses' Station layout, or hospital floor architecture that you find in your real-life clinical rotations. If you have already had experience within actual clinical settings, take a few moments to list the similarities and differences between the Canyon View virtual hospital and the real hospitals you have visited. There is considerable variation among hospitals in the United States, so think of *Virtual Clinical Excursions—General Hospital* as simply one type of hospital and take advantage of the opportunity to practice learning how, where, when, and why to find the information, medication, and equipment resources you need to provide the highest quality patient care.

The following icons are used throughout the workbook to help you quickly identify particular activities and assignments:

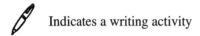 Indicates a reading assignment—tells you which textbook chapter(s) you should read before starting each lesson

Indicates a writing activity

Marks the beginning of an interactive CD-ROM activity—signals you to open or return to your *Virtual Clinical Excursions—General Hospital* CD-ROM

Indicates a continuation of CD-ROM activity instructions

Indicates questions and activities that require you to consult your textbook

Social Context of Nursing

Reading Assignment   The Nursing Profession (Chapter 1)
Legal and Ethical Context of Practice (Chapter 2)
The Health Care Delivery System (Chapter 4)

Patients: Paul Jungerson, Room 602
Darlene Martin, Room 613

Objectives

1. Identify the components of the health record in the context of the purpose and characteristics of documentation.
2. Identify examples of the documentation addressing standards of nursing practice.
3. Identify the members of the health care team in a patient's health record.
4. Locate information about legal/ethical issues in the patient's record.

Introduction

Paul Jungerson is a 61-year-old male admitted to the hospital on Friday to be prepared for surgery to resect (cut out) his cancerous colon and form a colostomy. His case is different from Ms. Martin, who had the surgical workup as an outpatient. Mr. Jungerson has a history of heart disease. You can review his records on the day of admission, the day of his surgery, and the first two days postoperative. You will visit Mr. Jungerson on his third postoperative day (Tuesday).

Darlene Martin is a 49-year-old female who has been experiencing irregular menstrual periods and an increasingly enlarged uterus. She has been diagnosed with fibroids. Due in part to a significant family history of endometrial cancer, she is being admitted for a total abdominal hysterectomy. You can review Ms. Martin's records on the day of her preoperative assessment (Thursday) and care for her on the day of her surgery (the following Tuesday).

Exercise 1—The Health Care Record

 This exercise will take approximately 90 minutes to complete.

 Read about documentation on p. 39 of your textbook.

 1. List the four characteristics of good documentation.

2. State the primary purpose of the patient record.

3. List the parts of the patient record in the order in which they appear on the tabs of the Charts at Canyon View Regional Medical Center. (*Hint:* Review the **Getting Started** section of this workbook if you need help.)

 Read about standards of practice on p. 9 of your textbook.

4. Define *standards of practice*.

5. List the titles of the six standards of care found in Appendix A of your textbook.

(1)

(2)

(3)

(4)

(5)

(6)

Note: You are about to log in for your first CD-ROM activity. You may want to answer all the questions from the textbook before you log in, or you can just stay logged in throughout the entire exercise. If the period of care ends before you have collected all the information you need, you can erase the data and log in again.

CD-ROM Activity

With *Virtual Clinical Excursions—General Hospital* Disk 2 in your CD-ROM drive, double-click on the **Shortcut to VCE** icon on your computer's desktop. Enter the Canyon View Regional Medical Center by clicking on the hospital doors. This takes you into the lobby; from there, click on the elevator. Inside the elevator, click on the floor directory panel to the right of the open door. Select button **6** since your first patient is on Floor 6. When the doors reopen, click on the **Nurses' Station** to enter the floor. Next, find and double-click on the **Supervisor's (Login) Computer**. Log in to care for Paul Jungerson at 07:00.

After listening to the Case Overview and reading the Preceptor Note, go to the Nurses' Station and access the patient's Chart. To do this, click on **Patient Records** on the upper left side of your screen and select **Chart** from the drop-down menu. Here you will be able to identify the elements in a patient's medical record. After you have reviewed Mr. Jungerson's Chart, return to the Nurses' Station and access the Kardex (click on **Patient Records**, then on **Kardex**). This is the best place to find the current physician orders and the nursing care plan.

Note: The Kardex is a summary of the key elements of an interdisciplinary plan of care. This plan of care is a working document that often is not part of the patient's permanent record. It may be kept in an actual Kardex file, placed in the patient's Chart, accessed from a computer, or located at a workstation outside the patient's room. Canyon View Regional Medical Center keeps a Kardex file on the counter of the Nurses' Station between the Electronic Patient Record (EPR) and the Medication Administration Record (MAR). As an alternative to using the drop-down menu on the left side of your screen, you may also click directly on the Kardex folder itself on the counter. *Remember:* Once you open the Kardex, you have access to *all* patients' Kardex plans—not just the patient for whom you are currently signed in. The Kardex is organized by tabs that match the patients' room numbers, so be sure to click on the correct tab for your patient on the right side of the opened Kardex.

The following activities will help you become familiar with the medical record and recognize the implementation of nursing standards of practice in the record.

→ Click on tab **602** and read Mr. Jungerson's Kardex.

6. Record the following information from Mr. Jungerson's Kardex.

Name of surgical procedure and number of postoperative days	
Can he have coffee with his breakfast?	
If he goes into cardiac arrest, what would you do? (*Hint:* Look at his code status.)	
Do you need to get him a urinal?	
What lab work is ordered for today? Does he need to be NPO until it is done?	

7. Which standards of care are addressed in the Kardex?

→ Return to Mr. Jungerson's Chart. (From the Kardex, click on the **Nurses' Station** icon in the lower right corner. You may then click on **Patient Records** and select **Chart**, or you can simply click on the stack of Charts on the counter of the Nurses' Station.) Inside Mr. Jungerson's Chart, review the History & Physical, Nursing History, and Progress Notes.

Remember: One of the standards of care is assessment. Part of your assessment is to review the patient's history and physical examination.

Note: Reviewing a patient record is like looking at a still photograph taken from the middle of a movie of the patient's life or like starting a novel in the middle. You need to know what brought Mr. Jungerson to this moment in time. The History & Physical tells you what has brought him to the hospital. The Progress Notes tell you what happened during his hospitalization. In the Nursing History you will find the patient's *usual pattern* functioning, and in Progress Notes you will find the patient's *current pattern* of functioning.

8. Below, list four problems from the History & Physical that might be important to Mr. Jungerson's nursing care in his postsurgery experience. *Hint:* You may not know all the medical terms, but you will probably spot some possible problems if you use your imagination and think about what it would be like to having surgery yourself and how it would feel to recover from a medication-induced state of unconsciousness (anesthesia). For each problem you identify, briefly explain how you think it will affect Mr. Jungerson's current care.

Problem	**How Do You Think It Will Affect His Current Care?**

Exercise 2—The Health Care Team

 This exercise will take approximately 30 minutes to complete.

 Review pp. 59-60 in Chapter 4 of your textbook.

 9. List the members of the health care team.

Review Mr. Jungerson's Chart and Kardex to find the members of the health care team who are caring for him. (*Hint:* Use the Kardex to determine what team members might be involved in his care, and then look at the Progress Notes and other sections of the Chart. Remember, all the health team members write in the same Progress Notes file.)

10. Below, list each member of Mr. Jungerson's health team (by occupation or role, not by name). Next to each member, identify what type of data or patient care issues that member recorded (or might record) in the Progress Notes.

Health Care Team Member	Type of Data and/or Patient Care Issues Recorded in Progress Notes

Click on the **Laboratory Reports** tab of the Chart. (*Remember:* The standard for assessment also includes the review of lab reports.)

11. For each diagnostic test listed below, record the most current results for Mr. Jungerson (from Tuesday). Compare his results with the normal values provided in column 2 and identify whether Mr. Jungerson's results were low, high, or within normal limits (WNL). Also briefly explain any significance of the test or results and list any action that needs to be taken.

Diagnostic Test	Normal Values	Results (Tues)	Comparison/Significance/Action
WBC	4.5–11		
Hemoglobin	12–18		
Hematocrit	36–52		
Glucose	60–110		
BUN	7–21		
Creatinine	0.5–1.2		
Prothrombin time (PT)	11–13		
Potassium	3.6–5.5		

Exercise 3—Ethical and Legal Issues

 This exercise will take approximately 20 minutes to complete.

 In Chapter 2 of your textbook, read about ethical and legal issues concerning patient rights. Pay specific attention to pp. 35-37.

 12. Define the following terms.

Advance directive

Do not resuscitate (CPR orders)

Informed consent

Confidentiality

 Search Mr. Jungerson's records to locate information about the issues listed in question 13.

13. Fill in the table below about Mr. Jungerson.

Issue	Where to Look	Data From the Record
Does the patient have an advance directive?		
Code status (Should you initiate CPR?)		
Informed consent		
Confidentiality		

CD-ROM Activity

Let's take a virtual leap in time to visit Mr. Jungerson during a later period of care. Return to the Nurses' Station and click on the **Supervisor's (Login) Computer**. Then click the **Supervisor's Computer** button (this will log you off). Next, select the **Nurses' Station** button and click on the **Login Computer** again. This time, log in to check Mr. Jungerson's status at 13:00. Open his Chart and review the Progress Notes. Look for entries that tell you what happened as a result of nursing care. You should be looking for assessment data—that is, descriptions of his wound, pain, or lung sounds. *Remember:* By assessing after care, nurses collect data for evaluation.

14. For each problem listed below, identify examples from the nurse's Progress Notes on Tuesday at 06:00 that address standards of practice for evaluating the problem.

Problem	Data for Evaluation (Tuesday 06:00)
Pain	
Breathing	
Nutrition	

Exercise 4—Comparison With a New Patient

This exercise will take approximately 20 minutes to complete.

 CD-ROM Activity

Now let's repeat the activities you just completed with a new patient. This time, you will visit Darlene Martin in the Ambulatory Surgery Unit before her surgery. Since you previously visited Mr. Jungerson *after* his surgery, you will be able to compare how much and what kinds of data you have about a patient at different points in the hospital experience.

If you are currently logged in, double-click on the **Supervisor's (Login) Computer** and sign off from your current patient and period of care. Click inside the elevator and go to the Surgery Department (Floor 4). When you arrive on the floor, click on the **Nurses' Station**; then double-click on the **Supervisor's (Login) Computer**. Sign in to care for Darlene Martin during the preoperative period of care (06:30–07:29). Return to the Nurses' Station and access Ms. Martin's Kardex.

15. Record the following information from Ms. Martin's Kardex.

Name of surgical procedure and number of postoperative days	
Can she have coffee with her breakfast?	
If she goes into cardiac arrest, what would you do? (*Hint:* Look at her code status.)	
Do you need to get her a urinal?	
What lab work is ordered for today? Does she need to be NPO until it is done?	

→ Access Ms. Martin's Chart and read the History & Physical.

16. Below, list three problems from Ms. Martin's History & Physical that might affect her postoperative nursing care. Explain how you think each problem will affect her care.

Data	**How Do You Think It Will Affect Postoperative Care?**

Review Ms. Martin's Chart and determine the members of her health care team.

17. Below, list the members of Ms. Martin's health care team (by occupation or role, not by name.) Next to each member, identify what type of data or patient care issues that member recorded (or might record) in the Progress Notes.

Health Care Team Member	Type of Data and/or Patient Care Issues Recorded in Progress Notes

→ Click on the **Laboratory Reports** tab in Ms. Martin's Chart.

18. For each test listed below, record Ms. Martin's prehospital laboratory results Compare her results with the normal values provided in column 2 and identify whether or not Ms. Martin's results are within normal limits. Also briefly explain any significance of the test or results and list any action that needs to be taken.

Diagnostic Test	Normal Values	Results (Tues)	Comparison/Significance/Action
WBC	4.5–11		
Hemoglobin	12–18		
Hematocrit	36–52		
Glucose	60–110		
BUN and	7–21		
Creatinine	0.5–1.2		
Prothrombin time (PT)	11–13		
Potassium	3.6–5.5		

Search Ms. Martin's records to locate information about the issues listed in question 19.

19. Fill in the table below about Ms. Martin.

Issue	Where to Look	Data From the Record
Does the patient have an advance directive?		
Code status (Should you initiate CPR?)		
Informed consent		
Confidentiality		

After her time in the Surgery Department, Ms. Martin is transferred to the Medical-Surgical Floor. Let's visit her there. Return to the Nurses' Station and click on the **Supervisor's (Login) Computer**. Then click the **Supervisor's Computer** button (this will log you off). Next, select the **Nurses' Station** button. Click inside the elevator and go to Floor 6. Once there, enter the Nurses' Station and click on the **Login Computer**. Sign in to see Ms. Martin at 11:00. Access her Chart and review the Progress Notes. Look for entries that tell you what happen as a result of nursing care. *Remember:* You should be looking for assessment data—that is, descriptions of the wound, pain, or the lung sounds. By assessing after care, nurses collect data for evaluation.

20. For each problem listed below, identify examples from th 12:00 Progress Notes on Tuesday that address standards of practice for evaluating the problem. *Remember:* This is the admission from PACU; therefore you are evaluating the effects of her surgery.

Problem	Data for Evaluation
Pain	
Breathing	
Nutrition	

A Framework for Nursing Practice

/○ℛᴆ **Reading Assignment:**   Caring and Clinical Judgment (Chapter 5)
Client Assessment: Nursing History (Chapter 6)
Assessing Vital Signs (Chapter 7)
Physical Assessment (Chapter 8)
Nursing Diagnosis (Chapter 9)
Planning, Intervening, and Evaluating (Chapter 10)
Documenting Care (Chapter 11)

Patient: Elizabeth Washington, Room 604

Objectives

1. Identify the major components from selected nursing theories.
2. Compare the elements of the nursing history with the medical history.
3. Collect data in each of the functional health patterns.
4. Write nursing diagnoses for a patient.
5. Plan for intervention and evaluation for a patient.
6. Identify where nursing process data are recorded.
7. Identify implementation of the standards for documentation in the health record.

Introduction

In this lesson you will identify the use of the nursing process from health records. Elizabeth Washington is a 63-year-old female who was admitted to the hospital following a motor vehicle accident (MVA). She sustained a fracture of the left acetabulum and was taken to the operating room for an open reduction and internal fixation (ORIF) of the fracture. During this lesson, you will care for Ms. Washington on her first postoperative day.

Patients with acetabular fractures often require an ORIF, especially those patients who also have displacement of the joint. The surgeon realigns or reduces the bones as precisely as possible to prevent the development of post-injury–related problems, especially arthritis. The bones are rigidly fixed with plates and screws to prevent future displacement and allow rehabilitation to begin as quickly as possible.

Early ambulation helps avoid some of the complications associated with these injuries. Because there are multiple variations in acetabular fractures, the surgeon should write specific orders for weight bearing and ambulation. In general, for 8 weeks the injured hip should bear no more than 30 pounds of weight. Physical therapy is designed to maintain muscle strength and range of motion during recovery. On the second day following surgery for an acetabular fracture, patients are usually able to get out of bed. Crutches must be used for 8 weeks following surgery, but by 12 weeks most people are able to walk unassisted. If they are otherwise in good condition, most people recover fully within 4 to 6 months and are able to resume recreational activities at that time. It may take a year for full recovery.

For some time after surgery, patients may continue to experience decreased sensation in a limb and/or difficulty or inability in moving part of the limb because of nerve damage secondary to the traumatic event or the surgery. Important branches of the lumbar and sacral nerves may be either stretched or torn, especially in the case of unstable pelvic fractures. The majority of patients do regain some sensation and function of the limb within 6 to 18 months after their injury. Avascular necrosis is a late complication resulting in the need for a total hip replacement. Provided that the hip can be properly aligned and fixed, 80% to 85% of patients can expect a good to excellent recovery following surgery.

Exercise 1—Assessing the Patient: History-Taking

 This exercise will take approximately 20 minutes to complete.

 Read about nursing theorists on pp. 74-76 of your textbook.

 1. Listed below are several important nursing theorists. Identify the major components of the nursing theory of each of them.

Lydia E. Hall

Ida Jean Orlando

Madeleine M. Leininger

Ann Boykin and Savina Schoenhofer

The following activity links with Exercise 2.

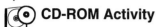 **CD-ROM Activity**

With *Virtual Clinical Excursions—General Hospital* Disk 2 in your CD-ROM drive, double-click on the **Shortcut to VCE** icon on your computer's desktop. Enter the hospital, click on the elevator, and go to Floor 6. When you arrive on the floor, click on the **Nurses' Station**; then double-click on the **Supervisor's (Login) Computer**. Sign in to care for Elizabeth Washington at 07:00. To familiarize yourself with Ms. Washington's condition, listen to the Case Overview and click on **Assignment** to read the Preceptor Note. Then return to the Nurses' Station. Before visiting Ms. Washington, access her Chart (click **Patient Records**; then select **Chart**). Review the History & Physical and Nursing History sections of the Chart.

You are now ready to visit the patient and perform a complete assessment. Return to the Nurses' Station, click on **Patient Care** (on the upper left side of your screen), and select **Data Collection**. This takes you to the sink area outside the patient's room. *Remember:* You must wash your hands before entering the room! Double-click on the sink and then click on the green curtain to the right of the sink. Once inside the room, click on **Initial Observations** and watch the interaction between the nurse and patient. Keep notes of any findings you want to remember. Continue the assessment by clicking on each of the buttons on the left side of your screen. When additional subcategories appear under the video screen, click on each of those buttons as well. Finally, click on each area of the 3-D body model (*Note:* as you move your cursor over the model, it rotates and the area under your cursor is highlighted. Click when the area you wish to assess is highlighted.) For each body area, a list of subcategories will appear under the video screen. Select them one at a time and make note of your findings. When you have completed the assessment, click on **Nurses' Station**. (*Remember:* You must wash your hands before leaving the patient's room!)

2. Consider the nursing theories you summarized in question 1. Based on what you know about Ms. Washington so far, which of those theories would you apply to her care? Why?

3. Define the following terms.

Critical thinking

Clinical judgment

Problem solving

Exercise 2—Nursing History

 This exercise will take approximately 30 minutes to complete.

 Read "Client Assessment: Nursing History" on pp. 100-103 in your textbook. Consider the questions that you might ask Ms. Washington to gather data for each functional health pattern.

 The following activities are linked with Exercises 1, 3, 4, and 5.

🔘 CD-ROM Activity

If you haven't already done so, enter Canyon View Regional Medical Center, go to Floor 6, and log in to care for Elizabeth Washington at 07:00. After reviewing your assignment, return to the Nurses' Station, open the Chart, and review the entire History & Physical and Nursing History sections. *Remember:* Ms. Washington was admitted on Sunday. Because it is now the day of surgery, you have more data about her condition.

4. List three differences you identified between the History & Physical and the Nursing History sections of the Chart.

   a.

   b.

   c.

5. Using the functional health patterns listed below and on the next two pages, briefly summarize the data the admitting nurse collected about Ms. Washington. (*Hint:* These findings are recorded in the Nursing History section of the Chart. You can also add any information you think is important from the History & Physical.)

Functional Health Pattern	Data From Ms. Washington
Health Perception- Health Management	
Nutritional-Metabolic	

Functional Health Pattern	Data From Ms. Washington
Elimination	
Activity-Exercise	
Sleep-Rest	
Cognitive-Perceptual	
Self-Perception–Self-Concept	
Role-Relationships	

Functional Health Pattern	Data From Ms. Washington
Sexuality-Reproduction	
Coping-Stress Tolerance	
Value-Belief	

Exercise 3—Making a Nursing Diagnosis

 This exercise will take approximately 20 minutes.

 Read pp. 181-183 in your textbook about the components of a nursing diagnosis. Also refer to the list of NANDA labels on pp. 179-181. Finally, review Chapter 8 (Physical Assessment) in relation to the problems listed below and on the next page.

CD-ROM Activity

If you aren't currently signed in, go to the Login Computer on Floor 6 and sign in to see Elizabeth Washington at 07:00. Your goal for this exercise is to develop nursing diagnoses based on what you know from the patient's records and physical assessment. (*Hint:* Look ahead to question 6 to guide your review.) First, review the Kardex plan of care.(Click on **Patient Records** and select **Kardex** from the drop-down menu.) Once the Kardex opens, remember to click on tab **604** (Ms. Washington's room number) to access the correct records. Review all three pages of the Kardex; then return to the Nurses' Station. Now access the patient's Chart and review the History & Physical, Nursing History, and Progress Notes as needed to complete question 6.

FYI: This is Ms. Washington's first day post-op from a surgical repair of a fractured acetabulum (ORIF). Here is a list of the problems the nurse would anticipate for this patient:
- Pain
- Respiratory complications (not as common with spinal anesthesia, but her lungs still need to be checked since she has asthma)
- Deep vein thrombosis (blood clots in the leg are common after hip fractures; the clot could break loose and go to her lungs)
- Risk for nerve damage causing urinary incontinence, impotence, foot drop, etc.
- Anxiety about moving and getting out of bed
- Poor tolerance for diet (anesthesia and pain medication can slow peristalsis, leading to abdominal distention, sometimes even nausea and vomiting)

- Difficulty with urination and bowel elimination (think about how you would manage this with a fractured hip)
- Surgical wound healing (it is likely that she has wound drains and may require dressing changes)
- Planning for rehabilitation after the hospitalization

6. For each functional health pattern listed below, develop a nursing diagnosis (in two parts: label and related factor) or indicate that the pattern does not apply to Ms. Washington.

Functional Health Pattern	Nursing Diagnosis	
	Label	Related Factor (r/t)
Health Perception-Health Management		
Nutritional-Metabolic		
Elimination		
Activity-Exercise		
Sleep-Rest		
Cognitive-Perceptual		
Self-Perception–Self-Concept		
Role-Relationships		
Sexuality-Reproduction		
Coping-Stress Tolerance		
Value-Belief		

Exercise 4—Planning for Interventions

 This exercise will take approximately 20 minutes to complete.

 In your textbook, read pp. 197-199 about establishing outcomes and p. 202 about the elements of an intervention.

 7. Now it is time to write outcomes and interventions for Ms. Washington. First, in the middle column below and on the next page, rewrite the nursing diagnoses you developed in question 6. Then, for each diagnosis, provide one outcome and one intervention.

Functional Health Pattern	Nursing Diagnosis	Outcome and Intervention
Health Perception-Health Management	Health-seeking behavior r/t expressed interest in working at recovery and returning to usual activities	Outcome: Intervention:
Nutritional-Metabolic	Imbalanced nutrition: less than body requirements r/t need for increased nutrients for wound healing	Outcome: Intervention:
Elimination	Ineffective urinary elimination r/t difficulty getting in the best position for urination	Outcome: Intervention:
	Risk for constipation r/t inactivity and constipating medications	Outcome: Intervention:
Activity-Exercise	Activity intolerance r/t postoperative cardio-vascular instability and pain	Outcome: Intervention:
Sleep-Rest	Risk for disturbed sleep patterns r/t change in usual environment	Outcome: Intervention:

Functional Health Pattern	Nursing Diagnosis	Outcome and Intervention
Cognitive-Perceptual	Acute pain r/t surgical repair of hip, first post-op day	Outcome: Intervention:
Self Perception-Self Concept	Moderate anxiety r/t pain and immobility	Outcome: Intervention:
Role-Relationships	Ineffective role performance r/t temporary inability to engage in usual activities	Outcome: Intervention:
Sexuality-Reproduction	Ineffective sexual patterns r/t temporary inability to engage in sexual activity, secondary to medical restrictions on position of hip and pain	Outcome: Intervention:
Coping-Stress Tolerance	Readiness for enhanced coping r/t expressed willingness to learn to cope with recovery	Outcome: Intervention:
Value-Belief	Readiness for enhance spiritual well-being r/t expressed interest in using minister as a source of support	Outcome: Intervention:

Exercise 5—Evaluating Care

 This exercise will take approximately 30 minutes to complete.

 Review Box 10-9 on p. 214 of your textbook.

 8. Write a list of questions you would ask yourself or Ms. Washington to evaluate the success of the nursing plan you developed in question 7. Use your imagination by thinking about your own health patterns and how you would manage with a fractured hip.

CD-ROM Activity

For each outcome and intervention you identified in question 7, search Ms. Washington's Electronic Patient Record (EPR) and the Progress Notes in her Chart to determine whether the data for evaluation have been recorded. (*Note:* To access the EPR, click on **Patient Records** and select **EPR**. Enter the password—**nurse2b**—and click **Access Records**.)

9. Listed below and on the next two pages are 12 sample outcomes appropriate for Ms. Washington's problems. Below each outcome is an intervention to achieve the outcome. For each pair, record the evaluation data (if any) you found in Ms. Washington's records to indicate whether or not the intervention was successful in achieving the outcome.

Outcome and Intervention	Ms. Washington's Evaluation Data
Outcome: Plans for completion of activities of daily living after discharge	
Intervention: The nurse will discuss obstacles to bathing, dressing, and grooming (e.g., maintaining alignment of hip, limited range of motion, standing at bathroom sink)	

Outcome and Intervention	Ms. Washington's Evaluation Data
Outcome: Lists three nutrients needed for wound healing and names foods she enjoys eating that will supply these nutrients **Intervention:** Assess patient's level of knowledge regarding nutrients for wound healing	
Outcome: Maintains a satisfactory (without incontinence or retention) pattern of elimination **Intervention:** Assess q2h for need to urinate (e.g., ask patient about feeling the urge to void; assess abdomen for signs of full bladder)	
Outcome: Maintains her usual pattern of bowel elimination (BM qod) **Intervention:** Administer the ordered stool softener at bedtime with a full glass of water	
Outcome: Is able to get out of bed without dizziness **Intervention:** Dangle at bedside before attempting to stand	
Outcome: Gets 6 hours of uninterrupted sleep tonight **Intervention:** Arrange medication schedule and vital signs to allow for 6 hours of uninterrupted sleep	
Outcome: Achieves pain control sufficient to allow her to participate in getting out of bed with physical therapy **Intervention:** Administer pain medication 30 minutes (for IV) or 45 minutes (for oral) before physical therapy	

Outcome and Intervention	**Ms. Washington's Evaluation Data**
Outcome: Maintain a positive attitude about getting out of bed with physical therapy Intervention: Explain and establish mutual goal setting about the level of pain control necessary for physical therapy	
Outcome: Plans with her husband and coworkers methods of compensating for her inability to perform usual roles (e.g., deciding which household tasks must be done) Intervention: Review limitations on activity in postdischarge period and compare with her usual tasks	
Outcome: Lists the restrictions on range of motion of her hip and the implications for sexual activity Intervention: Consult with physician/ physical therapist about the restrictions on range of motion and the expected length of restrictions; review the information with patient and give permission to talk about the implications for sexual activity	
Outcome: Lists the priority problems for which she will need a coping strategy Intervention: Assess the usual methods of managing the functional health patterns and physical barriers in the home; help the patient list modifications she will need	
Outcome: Participates in rituals or practices that are appropriate to her religion Intervention: Support her decision to call her minister; allow private time for them to visit	

Exercise 6—Documenting Care

 This exercise will take approximately 30 minutes to complete.

 In your textbook, read pp. 223-225 (about the types of entries) and pp. 230-232 (about the documentation formats).

 10. Identify the type of information to be included in each category of a SOAP note.

S

O

A

P

CD-ROM Activity

If you are not currently signed in, log in to see Ms. Washington on Floor 6 at 07:00. Open her Chart and read the Progress Notes.

11. Which of the following types of documentation do you think Canyon View Regional Medical Center uses?

Charting by exception

Focus charting

SOAP charting

Clinical pathways

→ Read the physician's progress note on Monday at 06:30. This note is an evaluation of Ms. Washington's postoperative status on the first day after surgery.

12. Evaluate the physician's entry for the following criteria. Answer yes or no for each criterion.

Legible

Dated

Timed

Signed

Clear

Absence of biased statements

Brevity

13. This physician's progress note indicates Ms. Washington's status in relation to problems that he is concerned about on her first day postsurgery. For each of the problems listed below, identify the data from the physician's progress note that evaluates the status of the patient.

Postsurgical Problem	Data From Progress Note
Pain	
Cardiovascular instability	
Ineffective breathing	
Bleeding or hemorrhage	
Nerve damage or vascular damage	
Bowel function	
Renal function	

➡ Practice entering data in a flow sheet by charting the data from question 13 in the Electronic Patient Record (EPR). (*Hint:* Refer to p. 23 in the **Getting Started** section of this workbook.)

When you have completed all the exercises for Ms. Washington in this lesson, click on **Clinical Review** on the left side of your screen. Follow the onscreen directions to take the quizzes. (*Hint:* Refer to pp. 25–26 in the **Getting Started** section for additional help.) You will be asked to select NANDA diagnoses and NIC interventions. The NANDA diagnoses may not be the same ones you selected. That is OK. Your diagnoses may still be appropriate for Ms. Washington. Even if you are not familiar with NIC interventions, you can make some intelligent guesses.

The Tools of Practice

 Reading Assignment: The Nurse-Client Relationship (Chapter 12)
Client Teaching (Chapter 13)
Managing Client Care (Chapter 14)
Nursing Research (Chapter 15)

Patient: Paul Jungerson, Room 602

Objectives

1. Reflect on your own communication style.
2. Identify therapeutic and non-therapeutic communication techniques.
3. Write a teaching plan.
4. Plan for delegation of a patient's care.
5. Identify the steps in planning nursing research for a simple problem.

Introduction

Paul Jungerson, age 61, has undergone repair for a disruption of a colon anastomosis and cre-
ation of a colostomy. An anastomosis is a surgical procedure in which two ends of the colon are
sutured together, usually after a segment of the colon has been cut out. A colostomy is a new
opening to the colon from the surface of the abdomen. Unlike normal elimination, in which
the sphincter controls the passage of stool, the stool is evacuated from an abdominal stoma.
Mr. Jungerson will need to manage establishment of a pattern of elimination through diet and
fluid management, as well as cleanliness, odor, protection of his skin, and wound healing.

 Exercise 1—The Nurse-Patient Relationship and Patient Teaching

This exercise should take approximately 60 minutes to complete.

In your textbook, read "The Therapeutic Relationship and Facilitating Effective Therapeutic
Communication" on pp. 242-250. Pay attention to information on the following topics:
• Verbal communication
• Non-verbal communication
• Paralanguage (nonverbal components of speech)

1. Below, describe and evaluate your personal style of communication. Refer to the textbook for prompts and descriptors of behavior you exhibit frequently. (*Note:* An example is provided for each communication type to get you started.) Comment on whether you think your communication techniques are effective or ineffective and why.

Description of Your Style	Effective/Ineffective

Verbal

(*Example:* Give advice)

Nonverbal

(*Example:* Lean toward people when they talk)

Paralanguage

(*Example:* Speak slowly in a soft voice)

2. Which communication techniques do you use naturally? (If you don't know, ask a friend or family member.) Record your answers under each subhead in column 1 below. How might patients interpret or misinterpret your verbal and nonverbal messages? How might patients interpret or misinterpret your usual paralanguage if they believed you were using paralanguage intentionally? (For example, if you typically speak quickly, a patient might conclude that you were impatient or hurried.) Answer these questions in columns 2 and 3. Finally, consider what alternatives you could try for your natural techniques; list these in column 4.

Techniques I Use Naturally	Interpretations	Misinterpretations	Possible (Alternative)
Verbal			
Nonverbal			
Paralanguage			

3. Consider your recent social interactions. In your everyday interpersonal communications, what goals do you hope to achieve? (*Example:* Organize family activities.)

4. How are these goals different from the goals of therapeutic communication in the context of the nurse-patient relationship? (*Hint:* Refer to p. 242 in your textbook.)

5. In the left column below, list the less familiar therapeutic techniques that you anticipate will be more difficult for you to use. In the right column, write specific suggestions to yourself to help you practice these techniques in preparation for interacting with patients in the hospital. Refer to pp. 250-253 in your textbook if you need assistance. This exercise will help you enhance the variety of your therapeutic techniques and will help you feel more confident and competent as you interact with patients.

Less Familiar Techniques   **How Can I Practice These?**

CD-ROM Activity

With *Virtual Clinical Excursions—General Hospital* Disk 2 in your CD-ROM drive, double-click on the **Shortcut to VCE** icon on your computer's desktop. Enter the hospital, click on the elevator, and go to Floor 6. When you arrive on the floor, click on the **Nurses' Station**; then double-click on the **Supervisor's (Login) Computer**. Sign in to care for Paul Jungerson at 07:00. To visit Mr. Jungerson in his room, click on **Patient Care** and select **Data Collection**. Wash your hands before entering the patient's room. Once inside, click on **Initial Observations** and watch the brief video segment, observing and evaluating the nurse's verbal and nonverbal techniques. Continue this evaluation as you click on **IV**, **Wound Condition**, and **Behavior**. For Behavior, you will need to click on each subcategory as well: **Signs of Distress, Needs, Support, Understanding,** and **Activity**. Use your evaluation to answer the following questions.

6. Below, describe the nurse's verbal communication, nonverbal communication, and para-language, using the descriptors on pp. 246-247 in your textbook as a guide.

Verbal communication

Nonverbal communication

Paralanguage (nonverbal components of speech)

7. Listed in the middle column below are statements or responses made by Mr. Jungerson during the Data Collection. Consider how you might respond to each statement and write your proposed verbal response (exactly as you would say it) in the right column. Indicate any paralanguage and/or nonverbal behaviors (in your personal communication style) to which you intend to pay particular attention.

Assessment Area	Mr. Jungerson's Statements	Your Response
Initial Observations	"Abdominal pain and cramping"	
IV	"No" (denies tenderness)	
Wound Condition	No response (does not report tenderness)	
Behavior Signs of Distress	"Surgery stressful . . . surprise, really . . . came pretty soon after the death of my wife."	
Needs	"Pain medication would be nice,"	
Support	"Yes, I'm happy about the move—I do miss my wife a lot—I have been able to make friends, yes."	
Understanding	"Yes, previous surgery cut my colon and then reassembled it, and my understanding is the ends have weakened and come apart. The surgery on Saturday, I hope, repaired that problem."	

8. Can you predict how Mr. Jungerson would have responded to each of your proposed thera-peutic responses? In a therapeutic relationship, what determines what you say next?

9. Indicate additional statements you could make to incorporate teaching into the interaction during the following assessments.

Assessment	Additional Teaching Statements
IV	
Wound Condition	
Behavior Signs of Distress	
Needs	
Support	
Understanding	
Activity	

→ Now, assess Mr. Jungerson's readiness for teaching at the beginning of *each period of care* (07:00, 09:00, 11:00, and 13:00). To do so, you will need to log out and sign in again for each separate period of care. (*Note:* If you choose to repeat a period of care, you will see a warning screen. If this occurs, click **Erase** and continue.) Each time you sign in, go to Mr. Jungerson's room and perform the assessments you conducted earlier for questions 6 and 7.

10. a. Complete the table below, indicating any cues you notice regarding Mr. Jungerson's readiness for patient teaching.

Time	Cues Regarding Teaching Readiness
07:00	
09:00	
11:00	
13:00	

b. What did you learn from this process?

11. Below, design an individualized teaching plan for Mr. Jungerson based on the following nursing diagnosis:

    Deficient knowledge r/t ostomy wound care and colostomy maintenance

    Goal: Patient will demonstrate appropriate care of ostomy site prior to discharge

    Your teaching plan must address the following three issues: what to teach, when to teach, and how to teach. Refer to Chapter 28 in your textbook for help.

What to Teach

    a. Your first step is to decide **what to teach**. Try to put yourself in Mr. Jungerson's place. What would you want to know if you had a colostomy? What are the "have-to-knows"?

When to Teach

    b. Now decide **when to teach**. Based on what you have learned and observed about Mr. Jungerson's readiness for teaching, What are the advantages and disadvantages of each time listed below? Refer to the assessments you made earlier in Mr. Jungerson's room for questions 6 through 10.

Time	Advantages	Disadvantages
07:00		
11:00		
13:00		

How to Teach

    c. Finally, you need to consider **how to teach**. What teaching strategies will facilitate Mr. Jungerson's learning?

12. Now that you have developed your teaching plan, how will you know that learning has taken place?

13. List the advantages and disadvantages of each of the following methods of evaluating whether learning has occurred.

Method	Advantages	Disadvantages
Patient takes written posttest		
Patient verbalizes skill		
Patient demonstrates skill		

14. What would be *essential* for you to include in your documentation of the patient teaching?

Exercise 2—Managing Patient Care

 This exercise should take approximately 30 minutes to complete.

 Read pp. 274-279 in your textbook.

 Now, think about various leadership styles you have encountered. Use the table below to complete the following steps:

- In the first column, list two individuals you know who have different leadership styles. They may or may not be in managerial positions.
- In the second column, list specific characteristics of each person. (*Hint:* Use the terms from pp. 274-279 in your textbook.)
- In the third column, identify what you think each characteristic indicates about the person's beliefs about his or her role, about his or her peers and subordinates, and about the organization in which the person is employed.

Individual	Characteristics	Beliefs About . . .
		Role:
		Peers:
		Subordinates:
		Organization:
		Role:
		Peers:
		Subordinates:
		Organization:

15. In your own words, define *responsibility* and *accountability*. Be sure you are able to distinguish between these two terms.

16. Briefly define the following terms and identify the purpose of each within a health care organization.

Philosophy

Mission statement

Goals

Objectives

Policies

Procedures

Standards

17. How are the concepts in question 12 related to risk management?

18. Describe briefly the three main steps involved in quality assurance.

Read "Patterns of Work," regarding methods of organizing nursing care, on pp. 279-280 in your textbook.

19. Describe the features of the following nursing care patterns (forms of nursing unit organization) in terms of risk management.

Functional nursing

Team nursing

Total patient care

Primary nursing

Review Box 14-3 (Steps in Effective Delegation) on p. 282 of your textbook.

Imagine that you are the registered nurse caring for Mr. Jungerson. At 07:00, you are informed that a beginning nursing student will be assisting you with his care. Which of the following activities would you be comfortable delegating to a fundamentals nursing student?

_____ Vital signs

_____ Bath

_____ Changing linens

_____ Assisting Mr. Jungerson to the bathroom

_____ Assessment of his wound

_____ Monitoring his intravenous therapy

_____ Serving his meals

_____ Teaching about his colostomy care

_____ Assessing his pain

20. What steps should you follow to ensure you delegate appropriately?

21. How will you evaluate whether or not the delegation of the task was appropriate?

22. At 08:30, the nursing student informs you that a coworker and friend of Mr. Jungerson is visiting and has offered to help him with his self-care and learning needs related to colostomy care. The student wants to delegate Mr. Jungerson's care to the friend so that she can leave to observe in the operating room. As the registered nurse, are you comfortable with the student delegating Mr. Jungerson's care to a significant other? Write a verbal response to the student exactly as you would say it.

Read Box 14-4 (Steps for Managing a Planned Change) on p. 282 in your textbook and review the steps for assessment of learning needs on pp. 262-265.

23. What does Client Learning Needs Assessment have in common with the nursing process?

24. What does nursing process have in common with the steps for managing a planned change?

Exercise 3—Nursing Research

 This exercise will take approximately 20 minutes to complete.

 Review Chapter 15 in your textbook.

 25. In your own words, describe the purpose of nursing research.

26. List the steps in the research process.

27. You and your peers in nursing school have decided to research whether there is a relationship between nursing school and stress. You have formulated your statement of the research problem (see completed step a below). Now complete the remaining steps in the research process (below and on the next page) as they relate specifically to this research problem.

    Statement of the research problem: Is there a relationship between nursing school and stress?

    a. Review of the literature (What topics would you look up?)

    b. Development of a theoretical construct:

    c. What is stress? Where does stress occur?

    d. What possible relationships could exist between nursing school and stress?

    e. Identification of variables:

    f. Clarification of operational definitions:

    g. Formulation of the research questions:

    h. Selection of a research strategy:

j. Collection of data:

j. Analysis of data:

k. Interpretation of findings:

28. What relationship does nursing research have to the steps for managing a planned change? (*Hint:* Refer to Box 14-4 on p. 282 of your textbook for assistance.)

The Well Patient Across the Life Span

Reading Assignment: Infancy Through Adolescence (Chapter 16)
The Young, Middle, and Older Adult (Chapter 17)

Patients: Maria Ortiz, Room 308
James Story, Room 512

Objectives

1. Identify growth and developmental milestones in pediatric patients.
2. Plan for diversional activities and parent education for pediatric patients.
3. Identify the developmental stage for adult patients.
4. Identify modifications in patient education and discharge planning related to the developmental stage of an adult.

Introduction

In this lesson, you will visit two patients, each representing a distinct age group: Maria Ortiz, 8 years old, admitted with an exacerbation of asthma, and James Story, age 42, admitted for renal failure. During your care, you will plan for modifications based on the various stages of growth and development.

Exercise 1—Infancy to Adolescence

 This exercise will take approximately 25 minutes to complete.

 Review pp. 305-312 in your textbook.

 1. For each age group, identify some of the key milestones for each area of development listed.

Infants (ages 0–1)

Physical

Sensory

Motor

Psychosocial

Cognitive

Moral

Toddlers (ages 1–3)

Physical

Sensory

Motor

Psychosocial

Cognitive

Moral

Preschoolers (ages 3–5)

Physical

Sensory

Motor

Psychosocial

Cognitive

Moral

School-age children (ages 6–11)

Physical

Sensory

Motor

Psychosocial

Cognitive

Moral

2. Read about preschoolers and school-age children on pp. 326-327 in the textbook. Then, in the left column below, circle the health teaching items you think would be important for an 8-year-old who is in the third grade.Provide a rationale for each decision.

Health Teaching Item	Rationale
Harmful effects of smoking	
Basic four food groups	
Establishing regular habits of exercise	
Fire safety	
Immunizations	
How to call 911	

 ## CD-ROM Activity

With *Virtual Clinical Excursions—General Hospital* Disk 1 in your CD-ROM drive, double-click on the **Shortcut to VCE** icon on your computer's desktop. Enter the hospital, click on the elevator, and go to the Floor 3. When you arrive on the floor, click on the **Nurses' Station**; then double-click on the **Supervisor's (Login) Computer**. Log in to care for Maria Ortiz at 07:00.

Return to the Nurses' Station and open Maria's Chart. Review the History & Physical and Nursing History. Once again, return to the Nurses' Station. You are now ready to visit Maria in her room. Click on **Patient Care** and select **Data Collection**. Wash your hands and enter the room. Inside, click on **Initial Observations** and watch the interaction between Maria and the nurse. Next, conduct an assessment of Maria's behavior (click on **Behavior**, then on each subcategory: **Signs of Distress**, **Needs**, **Support**, **Understanding**, and **Activity**). Make notes about her development.

Pay attention to Maria's mother for information to help you answer the questions in the next exercise.

3. Based on Maria's developmental age, determine whether or not you think each of the following health teaching items is appropriate for her. Why or why not?

Pathophysiology of her disease

Side effects of medications

Independent decision making about using her inhaler

How to manage participation in sports

What to tell her friends about her asthma

How to avoid allergens

Exercise 2—The Well Adult

 This exercise will take approximately 25 minutes to complete.

 In your textbook, read pp. 334-336 about adult developmental tasks.

 4. List the possible developmental tasks for a single working woman with an 8-year-old daughter.

💿 CD-ROM Activity

If you are still signed in to care for Maria Ortiz, return to the Nurses' Station and log out. Once you have signed out, enter the elevator and replace *Virtual Clinical Excursions—General Hospital* Disk 1 with Disk 2. Then click on button **5** to go to the Intensive Care Unit on Floor 5. Sign in to visit James Story at 07:00. As you did with Maria, review the History & Physical and Nursing History sections of Mr. Story's Chart. Next, go to his room and perform a full Behavior assessment. Take notes regarding his development.

5. Compare Maria's mother with Mr. Story, who is about the same age. List possible developmental tasks for a 42-year-old man with renal failure who has been on dialysis for a year. Remember that he has been married for 7 years. Use your textbook to help develop your own thoughts.

6. Now that you have met Mr. Story and know more about him, how does that change your perspective about his developmental needs. What data did you collect that would be helpful?

7. How can you help Mr. Story so that the necessary lifestyle changes have a positive effect on his stage of development?

Health Perception–
Health Management Pattern

 Reading Assignment: Health Perception (Chapter 18)
Health Maintenance: Lifestyle Management (Chapter 19)
Health Maintenance: Medication Management (Chapter 20)

Patient: Julia Parker, Room 608

Objectives

1. Distinguish among several models of behavioral change.
2. Consider the variety of factors affecting behavioral change.
3. Gather data from the patient record to plan for health management.
4. Gather data about a patient's lifestyle that pertains to health perception and health management.
5. Make decisions and plan nursing interventions for an individual patient's discharge planning and discharge teaching.
6. Develop a strategy for implementing a medication management plan with a patient.
7. Identify risk factors for injury (fall) in the hospital.

Exercise 1—Health Perception

 This exercise will take approximately 60 minutes to complete.

 Read about concepts and definitions of health on pp. 355-359 in your textbook.

 1. Briefly define the following terms.

Health perception

Health promotion

95

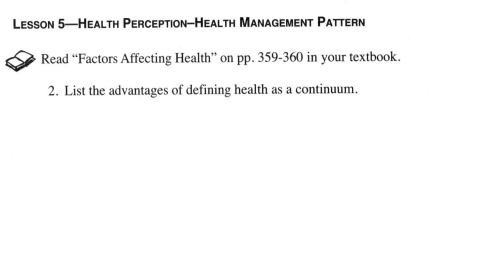 Read "Factors Affecting Health" on pp. 359-360 in your textbook.

2. List the advantages of defining health as a continuum.

3. Is the health continuum compatible with the concept of health as wellness and well-being?

Read "Factors Affecting Health: Assessment" on pp. 360-361 of your textbook.

4. List some questions you might ask your patients in order to collect data in each of the following areas (below and on the next page).

Questions Pertaining to Individual (Patient) Health

Questions Pertaining to Patient's Family Health

Questions Pertaining to Patient's Community Health

Questions for Focused Assessment: Health-Seeking Behaviors

 Read the case study on Mr. Oscar Kitchen in the boxes on pp. 367 and 369 of your textbook.

 5. Imagine that you are interviewing Mr. Kitchen. He informs you, "I stopped taking my medicine and resumed smoking because . . ." List several ways Mr. Kitchen might complete this sentence that would indicate he is a reasonable person who decided to stop taking his medication and/or to resume smoking.

 In your textbook, read "Concepts of Behavioral Change" on p. 367.

6. Define and differentiate the etic and emic dimensions of health.

Etic dimension

Emic dimension

Read "Models of Behavioral Change" on pp. 369-371 in your textbook.

7. Briefly identify the distinguishing features of each model or theory listed below.

Theory of Reasoned Action

Transtheoretical Model for Behavioral Change

Health Belief Model

Health Promotion Model

8. What concept seems to be central to each of the models in question 7?

Read "Factors Affecting Behavioral Change" on pp. 371-375 of your textbook.

9. In the first column below, list the nine factors identified in your textbook that affect behavioral change. In the second column, indicate whether each of these factors is under some control by the nurse, by the patient, by both the nurse and the patient, or by neither. Use the following system for marking: **N** for nurse only; **P** for patient only; **N and P** for nurse and patient. If the factor is not under the nurse's or the patient's control, write **No control**. For the purposes of this exercise, consider the nurse-patient relationship to be short-term, with a limited number of contacts.

Factor Affecting Behavioral Change	Under Any Control?
a.	
b.	
c.	
d.	
e.	
f.	
g.	
h.	
i.	

Read about interventions on pp. 378-383 of your textbook.

10. In the first column below and on the next page, list the interventions to motivate health behaviors and interventions to provide supportive care. In the second column, provide an example of each intervention for Mr. Kitchen.

Interventions	Individualized Interventions for Mr. Kitchen
a.	
b.	
c.	

Interventions	Individualized Interventions for Mr. Kitchen
d.	
e.	
f.	
g.	
h.	
i.	
j.	

Review the Key Principles of Chapter 19 on pp. 384-385 of your textbook.

CD-ROM Activity

With *Virtual Clinical Excursions—General Hospital* Disk 2 in your CD-Rom drive, double-click on the **Shortcut to VCE** icon on your computer's desktop. Enter the hospital, click on the elevator, and go to Floor 6. When you arrive on the floor, click on the **Nurses' Station**; then double-click on the **Supervisor's (Login) Computer**. Log in to care for Julia Parker at 07:00. Before you visit Ms. Parker, access her Chart and review the Nursing Admissions form in the Nursing History.

11. For each of the following sections of the Nursing Admissions form(below and on the next page), list any data or patient statements you found pertaining to motivation, locus of control, health perception, and self-efficacy.

Health Promotion

Nutrition/Metabolic

Activity/Rest

Perception and Cognition

Self-Perception

Coping and Stress Tolerance

→ Now go to Ms. Parker's room (*Remember:* Click **Patient Care**, select **Data Collection**, and wash your hands!) Inside her room, click on **Initial Observations**, then on **Behavior**, followed by each of the subcategories under the video screen. Observe the nurse-patient interactions for each segment. Listen specifically for the following: (a) patient's statements pertaining to motivation, locus of control, health perception, and self-efficacy and (b) the nurse's therapeutic verbal and nonverbal behavior. Bear in mind that the most influential factor in increasing the patient's participation in a therapeutic regimen is the relationship with the health care provider.

12. For each assessment area below and on the next page, write any statements by the patient (column 2) and any statements or nonverbal behavior by the nurse (column 3) that pertain to self-efficacy. (*Hint:* There is a lot of information here, and you may need to review each segment multiple times to ensure completeness and accuracy.)

Assessment Area	Patient's Statements	Nurse's Verbal and Nonverbal Behaviors
Initial Observations		
Behavior Signs of Distress		

Assessment Area	Patient's Statements	Nurse's Verbal and Nonverbal Behaviors
Needs		
Understanding		

13. During the 07:00–08:29 period of care, what nursing interventions did you observe that maximize self-efficacy in the patient?

14. As you review the nurse's verbal and nonverbal behaviors, what improvements can you suggest?

 Your supervisor requests that you participate on a committee to modify the Nursing Admissions form used in patient's Charts. Return to Ms. Parker's Chart and review this form in the Nursing History section as needed to answer the following questions.

 15. Identify the areas of the Nursing Admissions form that address self-efficacy.

16. What other questions can you suggest to the committee for addition to the Nursing Admissions form?

 If you are still logged in for Ms. Parker, go to the Supervisor's (Login) Computer and sign off.

Exercise 2—Medication Management

 This exercise will take approximately 30 minutes to complete.

Ms. Parker reported that she had experienced no medication side effects prior to her admission to Canyon View Medical Center. It is now Friday and your preceptor informs you that Ms. Parker will be discharged with the following medication orders:

Glyburide 3 mg PO qAM
Lisinopril 10 mg PO qd
Hydrochlorothiazide 25 mg PO qAM
*Docusate sodium 100 mg PO bid
*Coumadin 5 mg PO q 1700
*Nitroglycerin 0.4 mg SL, PRN for chest/back pain;
may repeat x 3 at 5-min intervals; if no relief after 20 min, get transport to ED

* Indicates a medication that is newly prescribed since admission

 Review the textbook's definitions of side effects and adverse effects on pp. 391-392.

 17. Next to each medication below and on the next page, list the side effects and any additional information you would like to give Ms. Parker. (*Hint:* Be sure to use a medication reference with nursing implications!)

Glyburide 3 mg PO qAM

Lisinopril 10 mg PO qd

Hydrochlorothiazide 25 mg PO qAM

Docusate sodium 100 mg PO bid

Coumadin 5 mg PO q 1700

Nitroglycerin 0.4 mg SL, may repeat x 3 at 5-min intervals.
If no relief after 20 min, get transport to ED.

 18. Your preceptor has identified the following nursing diagnosis for Ms. Parker: Risk for ineffective therapeutic regimen management. She has requested you to write a teaching plan for Ms. Parker's medications. Using Box 20-7 on p. 406 of the textbook, as well as a medication reference with nursing implications, write a list of interventions specific to Ms. Parker's medication regimen and learning needs.

19. Respond to each of Ms. Parker's statements below. You may use your medication reference as a resource, but remember that you would not be able to do so if the patient were right in front of you.

 a. "I know a little about Coumadin—my husband was taking that for 3 years, but he died anyway."

 b. "When I'm at home, can I take the Coumadin in the morning with the glyburide, just to keep it easy?"

 c. "I don't ever take Ambien at home for sleep, but once in a while, I take Benadryl to help me relax. Can I still do that with these medications?"

20. List the factors that indicate Ms. Parker is at risk for injury, particularly for a fall.

LESSON 6

Nutritional-Metabolic Pattern

 Reading Assignment: Promoting Healthy Nutrition (Chapter 23)
Restoring Nutrition (Chapter 24)
Maintaining Fluid and Electrolyte Balance (Chapter 25)
Promoting Wound Healing (Chapter 26)
Managing Body Temperature (Chapter 27)

Patients: Paul Jungerson, Room 602
Maria Ortiz, Room 308
James Story, Room 510
Elizabeth Washington, Room 604
Julia Parker, Room 608
Darlene Martin, Room 613

Objectives

1. Review normal nutrition with a patient.
2. Identify factors affecting a patient's nutritional status.
3. Make decisions about methods of nutritional assessment for a patient.
4. Plan for discharge dietary instructions.
5. Identify factors affecting a patient's fluid status.
6. Plan for implementation of the medical treatment plan.
7. Identify risk factors for wound healing for a patient.

 Exercise 1—Nutrition

 This exercise will take approximately 30 minutes to complete.

Review pp. 517-521 in your textbook. Read the case study of Joan on p. 517.

1. For each of Joan's questions (below and on the next page), write the response you would make if you were Joan's nurse. Use terms that would be understood by a "lay person" (i.e., someone not directly involved in the health care system).

   a. Joan asks, "What are the major components of food that I should know about?"

b. Joan says, "My nurse practitioner said I have to work more than twice as hard to burn fat calories as I do to burn protein or carbohydrates. What does the nurse practitioner mean?"

c. Joan asks, "What is nitrogen balance? Is that important?"

2. Based on the information you have, fill in the middle column below, providing specific factors that pertain to Joan. (*Note:* You will fill in Mr. Jungerson's column later.)

Factors Affecting Nutritional Status	Joan	Mr. Jungerson
Developmental stage		
Individual psychologic factors		
Physiologic factors		
Cultural, economic, and lifestyle factors		

CD-ROM Activity

With *Virtual Clinical Excursions—General Hospital* Disk 2 in your CD-ROM drive, double-click on the **Shortcut to VCE** icon on your computer's desktop. Enter the hospital, click on the elevator, and go to Floor 6. When you arrive on the floor, click on the **Nurses' Station**; then double-click on the **Supervisor's (Login) Computer**. Log in to care for Paul Jungerson at 07:00. Go to Mr. Jungerson's room and click **Initial Observations**. After you observe this video segment, conduct an assessment of his Behavior. Then return to the Nurses' Station, open Mr. Jungerson's Chart, and review the Laboratory Reports section.

Based on your initial observations and Mr. Jungerson's laboratory data, return to the table in question 2 and fill in Mr. Jungerson's column. What additional questions would you like to ask Joan and Mr. Jungerson? Add these to the table as well.

3. Consider the elements of nutritional assessment (lettered *a–e*) below and on the next page. If you were going to gather additional data for each patient, which method of assessment would you select? Provide rationales for your selections.

    a. Health (diet) history—Would you use the 24-hour recall, food frequency questionnaire, food diary, or household food consumption method?

For Joan:

For Mr. Jungerson:

    b. *Evaluation of food intake*—Would you use the food group method, nutrient composition method, or calorie count?

For Joan:

For Mr. Jungerson:

    c. *Physical assessment: Initial presentation, general appearance, and physical examination findings*—Based on their initial presentation, general appearance, and/or noteworthy physical examination findings, are these patients demonstrating any clinical signs of nutritional problems?

For Joan:

For Mr. Jungerson:

    d. *Physical assessment: Anthropometric measurements, particularly body mass index (BMI)*—What is each patient's BMI?

For Joan:

For Mr. Jungerson:

e. *Physical assessment: Diagnostic/laboratory tests*—For each patient, which laboratory test results are relevant to nutritional status?

For Joan:

For Mr. Jungerson:

4. If Mr. Jungerson asks you what he should eat when he goes home, what would you say?

Exercise 2—Nutritional Deficiencies

 This exercise will take approximately 20 minutes to complete.

 In your textbook, review Table 24-1 (Manifestations of Nutritional Imbalances) on p. 538.

 5. What conclusions can you make regarding the signs and symptoms of nutritional imbalances and the nursing implications?

 Review "Factors Affecting Nutritional Status" on pp. 539-541 in your textbook.

 6. Outline the risk factors affecting nutritional status.

CD-ROM Activity

For question 7, you will need to review the records of five patients in addition to Mr. Jungerson. For each patient, sign in for the 07:00 period of care and look for data that provide cues to possible nutrition problems. (*Note:* To access Maria Ortiz's records, you will need to switch from Disk 2 to Disk 1. If you need help, refer to p. 10 or p. 27 in the **Getting Started** section of this workbook.)

Review Table 24-1 (Cues to Possible Nutritional Problems) on p. 541 of your textbook.

    7. In the list under each of the following patients' names, underline any cues that you found in the patient's data, suggesting possible nutrition problems.

Mr. Jungerson

Anorexia, diarrhea, increased metabolic need, compromised immune system, less-than-normal nutrient consumption, low socioeconomic status, malabsorptive condition, polypharmacy, greater-than-normal nutrient consumption, muscle weaknesses in pharynx, soft palate or esophagus, psychological factors, reduced level of consciousness, nausea and vomiting

Ms. Parker

Anorexia, diarrhea, increased metabolic need, compromised immune system, less-than-normal nutrient consumption, low socioeconomic status, malabsorptive condition, polypharmacy, greater-than-normal nutrient consumption, muscle weaknesses in pharynx, soft palate or esophagus, psychological factors, reduced level of consciousness, nausea and vomiting

Ms. Washington

Anorexia, diarrhea, increased metabolic need, compromised immune system, less-than-normal nutrient consumption, low socioeconomic status, malabsorptive condition, polypharmacy, greater-than-normal nutrient consumption, muscle weaknesses in pharynx, soft palate or esophagus, psychological factors, reduced level of consciousness, nausea and vomiting

Ms. Martin

Anorexia, diarrhea, increased metabolic need, compromised immune system, less-than-normal nutrient consumption, low socioeconomic status, malabsorptive condition, polypharmacy, greater-than-normal nutrient consumption, muscle weaknesses in pharynx, soft palate or esophagus, psychological factors, reduced level of consciousness, nausea and vomiting

Mr. Story

Anorexia, diarrhea, increased metabolic need, compromised immune system, less-than-normal nutrient consumption, low socioeconomic status, malabsorptive condition, polypharmacy, greater-than-normal nutrient consumption, muscle weaknesses in pharynx, soft palate or esophagus, psychological factors, reduced level of consciousness, nausea and vomiting

Maria

Anorexia, diarrhea, increased metabolic need, compromised immune system, less-than-normal nutrient consumption, low socioeconomic status, malabsorptive condition, polypharmacy, greater-than-normal nutrient consumption, muscle weaknesses in pharynx, soft palate or esophagus, psychological factors, reduced level of consciousness, nausea and vomiting

Exercise 3—Fluid and Electrolyte Balance

 This exercise will take approximately 20 minutes to complete.

 Review "Functions of Body Fluids" on pp. 563-564 of your textbook.

 8. When is body fluid in a state of balance?

a.

b.

c.

d.

9. Describe briefly the characteristics of each fluid compartment.

Intracellular fluid

Extracellular fluid

Intravascular fluids

Interstitial fluids

Transcellular fluids

 Review the section on electrolytes in your textbook on pp. 564-566.

 10. Mr. Jungerson states, "My doctor keeps checking my electrolytes. Why is each of the electrolytes important?" In lay terms, write an explanation for the significance of each electrolyte (below and on the following page).

Sodium

Potassium

Calcium

Magnesium

Chloride

Phosphate

Review "Regulation of Fluid Balance" on pp. 568-569 in your textbook.

11. List the factors essential to fluid balance, along with their mechanisms of regulation.

Review "Factors Affecting Fluid Balance" on pp. 573-580 of your textbook.

12. Using the framework and headings below, outline the factors affecting fluid balance.

Lifestyle factors

Developmental factors
    Infants and children

        Adolescents and middle-aged adults

        Older adults

Physiologic factors

Clinical interventions

Review the clinical manifestations of acid-base imbalances (respiratory acidosis, respiratory alkalosis, metabolic acidosis, and metabolic alkalosis) on pp. 572-573 of your textbook.

13. For each of the following patient scenarios, identify the most likely acid-base imbalance: respiratory acidosis, respiratory alkalosis, metabolic acidosis, or metabolic alkalosis.

   a. Ms. Parker's nurse enters the hallway from the patient's room, saying, "She has no breathing and no pulse. Call a code!"

   b. Maria starts to think she is not able to breathe and says "I feel like I'm dying" as she hyperventilates.

   c. Mr. Story's wife informs you, "He's napping, even though he slept well last night." When you enter his room and approach his bed, you note that Mr. Story's respirations are deep and rapid. His breath smells "fruity," and you see an empty one-pound bag of chocolate candy next to the bed.

   d. Mr. Jungerson continues to vomit yellow-green gastric secretions. His doctor informs you, "I'm concerned that he's losing a lot of electrolytes in his vomitus, particularly potassium."

Exercise 4—Skin Integrity and Wound Healing

 This exercise will take approximately 30 minutes to complete.

 Review "Factors Affecting Skin Integrity and Wound Healing" on pp. 622-623 of your textbook.

14. For each patient listed below and on the next page, underline the factors currently increasing the patient's risk for impaired skin integrity and delayed wound healing. (*Note:* You may sign in to revisit these patients or review their records as needed.)

Mr. Jungerson and his colostomy site:

Personal hygiene, nutrition and fluid status, activity and exercise, smoking, substance abuse, age, immunosuppression, incontinence, hypoxemia, diabetes, infection, neurologic impairment, medications affecting protein synthesis and cellular growth

Ms. Martin and her hysterectomy incision site:

Personal hygiene, nutrition and fluid status, activity and exercise, smoking, substance abuse, age, immunosuppression, incontinence, hypoxemia, diabetes, infection, neurologic impairment, medications affecting protein synthesis and cellular growth

Ms. Parker and her femoral catheterization site:

Personal hygiene, nutrition and fluid status, activity and exercise, smoking, substance abuse, age, immunosuppression, incontinence, hypoxemia, diabetes, infection, neurologic impairment, medications affecting protein synthesis and cellular growth

Mr. Story and his thrombectomy/fistula removal site:

Personal hygiene, nutrition and fluid status, activity and exercise, smoking, substance abuse, age, immunosuppression, incontinence, hypoxemia, diabetes, infection, neurologic impairment, medications affecting protein synthesis and cellular growth

 ## CD-ROM Activity

For the next question, you need to visit Mr. Jungerson later in the morning. Log out for your current patient and period of care; then sign in again for Paul Jungerson at 11:00. After reviewing the Assignment, go to the patient's room and click on **Initial Observations**. Then conduct a full Nutrition and Behavior assessment.

 15. Based on Mr. Jungerson's current status, predict the course of his wound healing. What data did you use to reach this conclusion?

 Review Figure 24-3 (Decision Tree for Nutritional Assessment and Support) on p. 545 of your textbook.

 Let's jump ahead again in virtual time. Sign out of the current period of care and log on to care for Mr. Jungerson at 13:00. Review his Chart and the EPR through the course of his hospital stay, specifically tracking his temperature. (*Remember:* To access the EPR, click on **Patient Records**; then select **EPR**. Next, enter the password—**nurse2b**—and click **Access Records**. Once inside Mr. Jungerson's EPR, you will find his temperature data recorded in the Vital Signs summary. Use the blue arrows to scroll backward and forward through days and times.)

16. Dr. Anniston is considering supplemental nutrition for Mr. Jungerson. Can you predict how this patient will receive supplemental nutrition? Give your rationale.

17. Mr. Jungerson's temperature has varied through the course of his hospital stay. Plot his temperature on the graph below. (*Note:* Days and times are listed below each vertical line of the graph.)

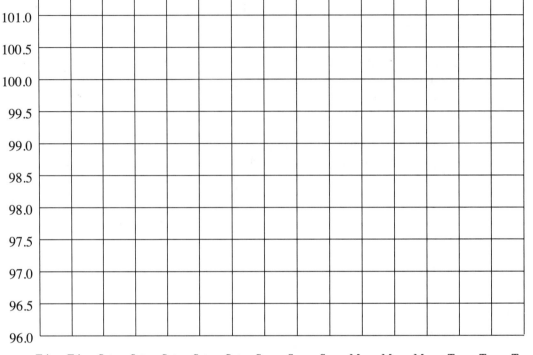

Fri	Fri	Sat	Sat	Sat	Sat	Sat	Sun	Sun	Sun	Mon	Mon	Mon	Tue	Tue	Tue
1200	1815	0000	1000	1415	1630	1800	0550	1419	2217	1019	1429	2205	0030	0925	1015

18. What advantage do you see to this method of documenting vital signs?

LESSON 7

Elimination Pattern

 Reading Assignment: Managing Bowel Elimination (Chapter 28)

Managing Urinary Elimination (Chapter 29)

Patients: Paul Jungerson, Room 602

Darlene Martin, Room 613

Objectives

1. Identify the patterns of urinary and bowel elimination for a hospitalized patient.
2. Plan for nursing interventions to meet the elimination needs of a hospitalized patient.

Exercise 1—Bowel Elimination

 This exercise will take approximately 45 minutes to complete.

Review pp. 665-668 in your textbook about the factors that affect bowel elimination patterns.

FYI: Mr. Jungerson has had a surgical procedure: diverting colostomy with Hartmann's pouch. He had surgery previously to remove a cancerous portion of his intestine. At the site of the anastomosis (where the two ends of the resected bowel were sutured together) he developed a leak. Because intestinal contents were entering the peritoneal cavity, he had pain and inflammation.

Hartmann's procedure is performed when a carcinoma of the rectum is found to be unresectable either because of local invasion or because the patient is unfit for a major resection. It may also be used in situations in which a primary anastomosis would be dangerous (e.g., severe perforating diverticulitis or a condition such as Mr. Jungerson's).

The lower end of the rectum is closed with sutures or staples and left in the abdomen (known as *Hartmann's pouch*). The upper end of the bowel is brought out as a descending colostomy. The residual rectum is thus completely nonfunctioning. However, its secretions still pass through the anus.

When a Hartmann's procedure is performed for inflammatory conditions, the bowel may be reconnected when local inflammation has resolved, which will be several months later. Whether Mr. Jungerson's colostomy is temporary or permanent, he will need to learn to manage bowel elimination in a new way.

CD-ROM Activity

With *Virtual Clinical Excursions—General Hospital* Disk 2 in your CD-ROM drive, double-click on the **Shortcut to VCE** icon on your computer's desktop. Enter the hospital, click on the elevator, and go to Floor 6. When you arrive on the floor, click on the **Nurses' Station**; then double-click on the **Supervisor's (Login) Computer**. Log in to care for Mr. Jungerson at 09:00. He is now 3 days post-op. Open the Chart and review Mr. Jungerson's History & Physical and Nursing History.

1. How do you think each of the factors listed below might affect Mr. Jungerson's bowel elimination? Provide a rationale that explains why each factor is or is not particularly relevant to Mr. Jungerson.

Factor	Rationale for Relevance
Personal habits	
Nutrition/fluids	
Exercise	
Culture	
Developmental factors	
Motor/sensory factors	
Medications	
Surgical procedure	

Review pp. 668-669 in your textbook regarding assessment.

2. Write five questions you would like to ask Mr. Jungerson to assess his bowel elimination pattern.

    a.

    b.

    c.

    d.

    e.

3. List the elements of the history and physical examination that are most pertinent to Mr. Jungerson's bowel elimination.

Read about nursing diagnoses on pp. 672-675 of your textbook.

4. List four nursing diagnoses for Mr. Jungerson related to the risk for constipation.

   a.

   b.

   c.

   d.

Return to the Nurses' Station, click on **Patient Records**, and select EPR. (*Remember:* Enter your password—**nurse2b**—and click on **Access Records**.) Inside the EPR, gather the most recent assessment data from the record. Finally, go to Mr. Jungerson's room and perform a complete physical assessment.

5. Record your data from the EPR and physical assessment below and on the next page.

Area of Assessment	Data Collected
Initial Observations	
Vital Signs	
IV	
Wound Condition	
Nutrition	

Area of Assessment	Data Collected
Behavior	
Head & Neck	
Chest & Back	
GI & GU	
Perineum & Rectum	
Upper Extremities	
Lower Extremities	

6. Based on the data you have collected, have you confirmed the tentative diagnoses you made in question 4? Rewrite your tentative diagnoses below and place an asterisk next to each one that is confirmed by your date.

a.

b.

c.

d.

7. Identify risk factors for constipation for Mr. Jungerson.

Return to Mr. Jungerson's Chart. This time, review the Physician Orders and his Medication Records.

8. Is there a laxative order? If so, why?

FYI: Mr. Jungerson's physician is not likely to order a laxative while he is in the hospital. It is preferable to train the bowel to a natural pattern of elimination. Some physicians will allow the use of laxatives, whereas others will not. Another factor is whether the colostomy is in the ascending, transverse, or descending colon. Strong laxatives have the potential for excess loss of fluid and electrolytes. Bulk laxatives can remain in the colon and cause an impaction. Lubricant laxatives may be the best choice.

9. Sometimes, for a patient without a bowel condition you may see a physician's order that simply says "laxative of choice." In this case, what type of medication would you choose? Discuss the advantages and/or drawbacks of each of the three medication types listed below.

Laxative

Stool softener

Bulk-forming laxative

10. What specific areas of care would be included in colostomy care. What function of the colon is lost?

Exercise 2—Urinary Elimination

 This exercise will take approximately 40 minutes to complete.

 In your textbook, review pp. 698-699 about assessment of urinary elimination.

 11. Define the following terms.

Urge incontinence

Stress incontinence

Urinary retention

FYI: In a few minutes, you will switch patients and begin caring for Darlene Martin. Ms. Martin is having a total abdominal hysterectomy and bilateral salpingo-oophorectomy (TAH-BSO). *Total hysterectomy* means removal of the uterus and cervix. *Abdominal* means that the surgical approach is through an abdominal incision rather than through the vagina. *Bilateral oophorectomy* means removal of both ovaries. It is reasonable to remove the ovaries because Ms. Martin may be close enough to menopause that her ovaries are not functioning anyway; also she has a cyst on one ovary. Her uterus is the size it would normally be at 14 weeks of pregnancy, which may be one reason the surgeon is choosing an abdominal approach.

A fibroid tumor in the uterus can cause pressure on the bladder, resulting in urge incontinence or stress incontinence. When a surgeon is working in the abdomen, there is risk for nicking the ureters or bladder, especially when the bladder is full. Performing a hysterectomy requires working in close proximity to the bladder in a small space. Postoperative edema in the pelvis can further disrupt bladder function. A Foley catheter is frequently inserted to drain the bladder during surgery and to prevent postoperative urinary retention.

12. Write one question you would ask Ms. Martin in each of the categories below.

History of urinary dysfunction

Usual pattern of elimination

Past medical history

Presenting problem

13. Which of the following components (below and on the next page) of the physical examination would be important for Ms. Martin? Why?

Integumentary

Neuromuscular

Abdominal

Urinary retention

Bowel elimination

14. Identify the purpose of each diagnostic test listed below and on the next page. In the far right column, indicate whether or not each is a simple test to verify renal function.

Diagnostic Test	Purpose	Simple Test to Verify Renal Function? (Yes or No)
Urinalysis		
Urine culture		
Serum creatinine		
Blood urea nitrogen		

Diagnostic Test	Purpose	Simple Test to Verify Renal Function? (Yes or No)
Cystoscopy		
Urodynamic tests		
Imaging		

15. Based on what you know so far about Ms. Martin, what would be the rationale for intake and output measurement in her case?

CD-ROM Activity

To continue this exercise, you need to visit Darlene Martin on Floor 4.
If you are currently logged in for Mr. Jungerson, follow these instructions:
- Return to the Nurses' Station and double-click on the **Supervisor's (Login) Computer**. At the Warning screen, select the **Supervisor's Computer** button. You are now logged out.
- Now click inside the elevator and go to Floor 4. Once there, sign in to visit Darlene in the PACU at 09:30.
If you do not already have the software running, follow these instructions:
- With *Virtual Clinical Excursions—General Hospital* Disk 2 in your CD-ROM drive, double-click on the **Shortcut to VCE** icon on your computer's desktop. Enter the hospital, click on the elevator, and go to Floor 4. Go to the Login Computer and sign in to care for Darlene Martin in the PACU after her surgery.

Once you have signed in to visit Ms. Martin in the PACU, open her Chart and review these sections: History & Physical, Nursing History, Laboratory Reports, and Progress Notes.

16. Do Ms. Martin's laboratory results confirm good kidney function? Explain.

→ Go to Ms. Martin's room in the PACU and perform a complete physical assessment.

17. Below and on the next page, chart the data you collected in Ms. Martin's room.

Area of Assessment	Data
Initial Observations	
Vital Signs	
IV	
Wound Condition	
Nutrition	
Behavior	
Head & Neck	
Chest & Back	
Perineum & Rectum	

Area of Assessment	Data
GI & GU	
Upper Extremities	
Lower Extremities	

18. Do you anticipate any postoperative urinary elimination problems for this patient with TAH? Explain.

19. How would you prevent or manage this problem?

Activity-Exercise Pattern

 Reading Assignment: Managing Self-Care Deficit (Chapter 30)
Restoring Physical Mobility (Chapter 31)
Preventing Disuse Syndrome (Chapter 32)
Supporting Respiratory Function (Chapter 33)
Supporting Cardiovascular Function (Chapter 34)

Patients: James Story, Room 512
Elizabeth Washington, Room 604
Maria Ortiz, Room 308
Julia Parker, Room 608

Objectives

1. Assess and plan for interventions to meet the need for hygiene.
2. Assess and plan for interventions to increase the mobility of a patient.
3. Assess and plan for interventions to prevent disuse syndrome for a patient.
4. Assess and plan for interventions to support the respiratory function of a patient.
5. Assess and plan for interventions to support the cardiovascular function of a patient.

Exercise 1—Hygiene

This exercise will take approximately 30 minutes to complete.

James Story, age 42, came to the emergency department complaining of shortness of breath, increasing weakness with a tingling sensation in his extremities, nausea, recent onset of diarrhea, lower leg edema, and a significantly edematous right arm. Mr. Story has type I (insulin–dependent) diabetes mellitus and has been undergoing hemodialysis treatment for almost a year. He also has chronic renal failure.

FYI: Chronic renal failure, a possible complication of diabetes mellitus, is an irreversible progressive reduction of functioning renal tissue. Symptoms of uremia develop when the output is less than 20 ml/hour. BUN and creatinine levels are elevated. Potassium level is also elevated because the kidneys are critical to the excretion of excess potassium. Anemia may develop because the kidneys produce erythropoietin, which stimulates the production of red blood cells. Fluid accumulates in the body, resulting in edema.

Symptoms of chronic renal failure include fatigue, weakness, and cold intolerance; anorexia, nausea, and vomiting; bitter metallic or salty taste; fetid, fishy breath; constipation; decreased resistance to infection; accumulation of medication with risk for toxicity; cardiovascular complications; pulmonary edema; changes in the bones; dry skin, pruritus from calcium deposited on skin; orange, green, or gray color; brittle hair that tends to fall out; peripheral neuropathy; inability to concentrate, short attention span, and impaired reasoning.

Hemodialysis is the removal of waste products from the blood by ultrafiltration and diffusion. The blood is channeled from the body through a dialysis machine by which wastes, fluid, medications, and electrolytes are removed through a semipermeable membrane. A fistula is surgically created from an artery to a vein to have an easy access site to insert the dialysis cannula. Over time the fistula grows from arterial pressure and a bruit can be felt and heard at the site. There is risk for blood clotting at the site of the fistula.

 Read about factors affecting the need for hygiene and about assessing the need for hygiene on pp. 735-736 in your textbook.

 1. Think about how each of the factors listed below might affect Mr. Story's need for hygiene. In the right column list information you would need to gather regarding each factor to assess this need. (*Hint:* You may include data that would be found in the patient's records or information you would obtain directly from Mr. Story.)

Factor	Relevant Information to Assess Need for Hygiene
Personal habits	
Nutrition/fluids	
Exercise	
Culture	
Developmental factors	
Motor/sensory factors	
Medications	
Surgical procedure	

2. Write five questions that you would like to ask Mr. Story to assess his hygiene needs.

   a.

   b.

   c.

   d.

   e.

CD-ROM Activity

With *Virtual Clinical Excursions—General Hospital* Disk 2 in your CD-ROM drive, double-click on the **Shortcut to VCE** icon on your computer's desktop. Enter the hospital, click on the elevator, and go to Floor 5. When you arrive on the floor, click on the **Nurses' Station**; then double-click on the **Supervisor's (Login) Computer**. Log in to care for Mr. Story at 09:00.

3. Go to Mr. Story's room and conduct a full assessment. Record your data below and on the next page.

Area of Assessment	Data Collected
Initial Observations	
Vital Signs	
IV	
Wound Condition	
Nutrition	

Area of Assessment	Data Collected
Behavior	
Head & Neck	
Chest & Back	
GI & GU	
Perineum & Rectum	
Upper Extremities	
Lower Extremities	

4. In each of the following areas, what data are relevant to providing hygiene to Mr. Story?

Age

Developmental stage

Medical diagnosis

Activity limitations

Ability to perform self-care

5. Which of the following types of bath would you provide for Mr. Story?

_____ Complete bed bath

_____ Partial assistance

_____ Partial bath

_____ Shower

_____ Tub

6. What was the basis for your decision in question 5?

7. What special considerations would you make in providing hygiene to Mr. Story?

Exercise 2—Physical Mobility

This exercise will take approximately 40 minutes to complete.

In this exercise you will be visiting Elizabeth Washington. She is a 63-year-old patient who was admitted following an auto accident in which she fractured her hip. She has a history of hypertension and asthma. You previously worked with Ms. Washington if you completed Lesson 2. In that case, you may want to return to Lesson 2 and review the FYI note about her hip fracture.

FYI: The surgeon has ordered total hip precautions on Ms. Washington. Although these may vary somewhat with different surgeons, the following precautions are generally included:
- Do not cross one leg over the other; keep knees apart.
- Do not flex the hip more than 90° when putting on shoes and stockings. Use extenders or have help.
- Do not sit continuously for longer than 1 hour.
- Do not sit in low, reclining, or rocking chairs that would require flexion of more than 90°.
- Use a raised toilet seat.
- Place a pillow between knees when lying down.

In your textbook, review about factors affecting physical mobility and about assessment of physical mobility on pp. 770-773 and 777-780.

8. Think about how each of the factors listed below might affect Ms. Washington's need for mobility. In the right column list information you would need to gather regarding each factor to assess this need. (*Hint:* You may include data that would be found in the patient's records or information you would obtain directly from Ms. Washington.)

Factor	Relevant Information to Assess Need for Mobility
Personal habits	
Nutrition/fluids	
Exercise	
Culture	
Environmental factors	
Developmental factors	
Motor/sensory factors	
Medications	
Surgical procedure	

9. List five questions that you would like to ask Ms. Washington about her need for mobility.

a.

b.

c.

d.

e.

CD-ROM Activity

If you are still logged in for Mr. Story, log out and sign in to care for Ms. Washington at 09:00. If you do not already have the software running, insert *Virtual Clinical Excursions—General Hospital* Disk 2 in your CD-ROM drive, double-click on the **Shortcut to VCE** icon on your computer's desktop. Enter the hospital, click on the elevator, and go to Floor 6. When you arrive on the floor, click on the **Nurses' Station**; then double-click on the **Supervisor's (Login) Computer**. Log in to care for Ms. Washington at 09:00. From the Nurses' Station, click on **Patient Care** and select **Data Collection**. Wash your hands and enter the patient's room. Once inside, perform a complete assessment.

10. Record your findings from the assessment of Ms. Washington below and on the next page.

Area of Assessment	Data Collected
Initial Observations	
Vital Signs	
IV	
Wound Condition	
Nutrition	

Area of Assessment	Data Collected
Behavior	
Head & Neck	
Chest & Back	
Perineum & Rectum	
GI & GU	
Upper Extremities	
Lower Extremities	

→ Return to the Nurses' Station and open Ms. Washington's Chart.

11. What is the physician's order for activity?

12. Is Ms. Washington allowed to bear weight on the affected limb?

13. How will you get her out of bed?

14. What safety precautions will you use when you ambulate Ms. Washington?

Exercise 3—Disuse Syndrome

 This exercise will take approximately 40 minutes to complete.

 In this exercise you will continue with the care of Elizabeth Washington. This time you will review Ms. Washington's case for the risk for disuse syndrome.

 In your textbook read about the effects of immobility on pp. 802-807.

 CD-ROM Activity

If you are still signed in, return to the Nurses' Station and log out. Then return to the Login Computer and sign in to care for Ms. Washington at 11:00. *Note:* If you do not already have the software running, insert Disk 2 and follow instructions for the first CD-ROM Activity (p. 43 of this workbook.) Review your data from Exercise 2 of this lesson about Ms. Washington. Also, return to the Chart to gather more details from her History & Physical. (*Remember:* At this time of day, the nurse performs only those assessments that need to be done more often than q4h.)

 15. Consider how the factors listed below might affect Ms. Washington's risk for disuse syndrome. Explain why each factor is, or is not, particularly relevant to this risk.

Factor	Rationale for Relevance
Inactivity and immobility	
Musculoskeletal	
Integumentary	
Cardiovascular	
Respiratory	
Gastrointestinal	
Genitourinary	

16. For each risk listed below and on the next page, identify an intervention that you would like to implement as a preventative measure for Ms. Washington.

Specific Risk	Nursing Intervention
Risk for pneumonia	
Risk for deep vein thrombosis	

Specific Risk	Nursing Intervention
Risk for muscle atrophy in affected leg	
Risk for osteoporosis	
Risk for foot drop in affected limb	

➡ Ms. Washington is currently having an asthma attack. Go to her room to perform an assessment. (*Remember:* You did a thorough assessment in the previous period of care. At this time, you need to carefully consider your priorities and focus only on those areas of concern.)

17. Use the table below to record your priority data from the assessment of Ms. Washington. If you did not collect data for an area, indicate why (e.g., Not a priority).

Area of Assessment	Data Collected
Initial Observations	
Vital Signs	
IV	
Wound Condition	
Nutrition	
Behavior	
Head & Neck	
Chest & Back	
GI & GU	
Upper Extremities	
Lower Extremities	

18. Do you think Ms. Washington's risk for disuse syndrome is high, medium, or low?

19. How will you assess for and prevent the effects of bed rest?

Exercise 4—Respiratory Function

This exercise will take approximately 30 minutes to complete.

Shortly, you will sign in to care for Maria Ortiz. Questions 20 through 24 will provide information you need to follow Maria's case.

20. What is asthma?

21. What is SpO_2? (*Note:* Your textbook calls it *oxygen saturation*.) How is this vital sign measured at the bedside? Do you think this will be frightening to Maria? Why?

22. What does it mean when you hear wheezes in the lungs? When someone is having an asthma attack, what does it mean if the wheezes disappear, but the person is still having difficult breathing?

23. Identify the classification and purpose of the medications below in the treatment of asthma.

Medication	Classification	Purpose
Solumedrol 30 mg IV q6h		
Albuterol nebulizer		
Tylenol		

24. List the signs and symptoms of oxygen deprivation for each area of assessment.

 CD-ROM Activity

If you are currently logged in for another patient, sign out and return to the elevator. With *Virtual Clinical Excursions—General Hospital* Disk 1 in your CD-ROM drive, go to Floor 3. When you arrive on the floor, click on the **Nurses' Station**; then double-click on the **Supervisor's (Login) Computer**. Log in to care for Maria Ortiz at 11:00. Review Maria's EPR for today. (*Remember:* The password is **nurse2b**.) Next, access her Chart and review these sections: History & Physical, Nursing History, and Progress Notes.

25. Record the summary of what happened to Maria at 10:35 today.

Read about factors affecting respiratory function on pp. 838-842 of your textbook.

26. From Maria's History & Physical and Nursing History, record any information relevant to respiratory function in the following categories.

Factor	Data Relevant to Respiratory Function
Personal habits	
Nutrition/fluids	
Exercise	
Environmental factors	
Culture factors	
Developmental factors	
Physiologic factors	
Medications	

27. What questions would you like to ask Maria about factors affecting her respiratory function? For each factor listed below, write a question to ask Maria, along with a rationale for its relevance to respiratory function.

Factors	Questions to Ask and Why They Are Relevant
Personal habits	
Nutrition/fluids	
Exercise	
Environmental factors	
Culture factors	
Developmental factors	
Physiologic factors	
Medications	

→ Now go to Maria's room and collect data from the physical assessment as needed to complete question 28.

28. In the table below, record the assessment data collected during Maria's asthma attack (in column 2) and the current assessment data (in column 3). (*Hint:* Information about Maria's asthma attack can be found in the Preceptor Note provided to you when you signed in for this period of care. If you need to review that note, return to the Nurses' Station, click on **Patient Care,** and select **Case Overview** from the drop-down menu. Listen to the overview and then click on **Assignment** to read the Preceptor Note.)

Area of Assessment	Data During Attack	After Attack Is Subsiding
Initial Observations		
Vital Signs		
IV		
Wound Condition		
Nutrition		
Behavior		
Head & Neck		
Chest & Back		
GI & GU		
Upper extremities		
Lower extremities		

Exercise 5—Cardiovascular Function

 This activity will take approximately 30 minutes to complete.

FYI: Julia Parker, age 51, has suffered a myocardial infarction. She presented to the emergency department with indigestion and midback pain. She has a history of hypertension and asthma.

 29. Define the following terms.

Angina pectoris

Myocardial infarction

Dysrhythmia

Hypertension

Cardiac enzymes—LDH, CPK-MB, treponin

FYI: Ms. Parker has had an angioplasty. In this procedure a catheter is inserted in the femoral artery and threaded to the coronary arteries at the site of obstruction of the coronary artery. A balloon on the tip of the catheter is inflated to compress the obstruction and open the artery. The femoral site of the arterial puncture must be closely monitored for bleeding. A sandbag is used to compress the puncture site until hemostasis is achieved. Because of the pressure in the artery and the size of the puncture, the sand bag is left in place for an extended period of time. The patient must keep the leg extended and still until there is no danger of bleeding. Women are more likely to have atypical chest pain when they have a myocardial infarction. Ms. Parker's chest pain is atypical.

30. Ms. Parker is receiving the medications listed below and on the next page. Using a drug reference with nursing implications, give the classification of each medication and indicate its specific purpose for Ms. Parker's condition.

Medication	Classification	Purpose for Ms. Parker
Glyburide		
Hydrochlorathiazide		
Lisinopril		
Enoxaparin		

ASA

Acetaminophen

NTG

MS

Zolpidem tartrate

Ducosate sodium

In your textbook, review factors affecting cardiac function and assessment on pp. 889-897.

31. For each factor listed below, identify specific examples that may be relevant to Ms. Parker's cardiovascular function.

Factor	Examples Relevant to Cardiovascular Function
Risk factors	
Physiological factors	
Cultural and lifestyle factors	
Psychological factors	

32. Write questions you would like to ask Ms. Parker to assess her cardiovascular function.

CD-ROM Activity

If you are currently logged in, return to the Nurses' Station and sign out on the Login Computer. Then, with Disk 2 in your CD-ROM drive, enter the elevator and go to Floor 6. Access the Login Computer there and sign in to care for Julia Parker at 11:00. Go to her room to conduct an assessment. (*Remember:* You would not perform a complete physical assessment at this time. You need to focus your assessment on priority areas.)

33. Below and on the next page, enter the findings from your focused assessment of Ms. Parker.

Area of Assessment	Data Collected
Initial Observations	
Vital Signs	
IV	
Wound Condition	
Nutrition	

Area of Assessment	Data Collected
Behavior	
Head & Neck	
Chest & Back	
GI & GU	
Upper Extremities	
Lower Extremities	

34. What action do you think the nurse should take based on your assessment findings?

35. What do you think is happening to Ms. Parker?

Sleep-Rest Pattern

 Reading Assignment: Managing Sleep and Rest (Chapter 35)

Patients: Elizabeth Washington, Room 604
Julia Parker, Room 608
Darlene Martin, Room 613
James Story, Room 512

Objectives

1. Assess and plan for interventions to meet a patient's needs for sleep and rest.

Exercise 1—Rest and Sleep

This exercise will take approximately 45 minutes to complete.

 Review the case study of Ms. Emma Weiss on p. 916 of your textbook.

FYI: Although your patients may believe that rest and sleep are needed to achieve and maintain optimal health, they may not possess knowledge of normal rest requirements or normal sleep needs. It is often beneficial for patients to receive information about baseline rest and sleep requirements so that they can have language and concepts to be able to describe what rest and sleep needs are not being met in the hospital. (Often, nurses and other health care providers simply chart "The patient slept well" without further assessment or description.)

In addition, nursing assessment forms often do not solicit the detailed information you would like for describing a patient's baseline sleep pattern to compare with the patient's in-hospital (or current) pattern. Ms. Emma Weiss, the textbook's outpatient patient visiting her health mainte-nance organization, describes her symptoms and has arrived at a conclusion and a desired inter-vention ("sleeping pill") but may not be able to describe her usual sleep/rest pattern versus her current sleep/rest pattern, despite the fact that she certainly recognizes there is a problem.

 Review Concepts of Rest and Sleep on pp. 916-918 of your textbook.

Ms. Weiss is very interested in normal rest and sleep patterns and would like your assistance in creating some "bulleted lists" so that she can teach her family members.

1. List some characteristics of normal rest.

2. List some characteristics of normal sleep.

3. List some characteristics of rapid eye movement (REM) sleep.

4. List some characteristics of non-rapid eye movement (non-REM) sleep.

5. List some characteristics of normal sleep cycles.

6. Describe the functions of sleep.

7. List the regulators of normal sleep.

Review Sleep Pathologies on pp. 918-921 of your textbook.

8. Define the following three major sleep disorder categories and list examples for each.

Dyssomnia

Parasomnia

Medical-psychiatric sleep disorders

9. Of the three sleep disorders you defined in question 8, which do you think are most common in the general (nonhospitalized) population?

10. Which sleep disorders do you think nurses can impact most directly?

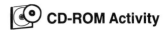 **CD-ROM Activity**

Consider your patients at Canyon View—particularly Ms. Parker, Ms. Martin and Ms. Washington—and the factors that may be affecting their rest and sleep. One at a time, sign in for these patients at 07:00 and review the History & Physical and Nursing History sections of their Charts. Look for data related to the factors listed in the table in question 11.

 Note: If you've already worked with any of these patients in previous exercises, go back and review your notes.

11. Use the table below to record your findings related to sleep and rest for Ms. Martin, Ms. Parker, and Ms. Washington.

	Ms. Parker	Ms. Martin	Ms. Washington
Nutrition pattern			
Exercise			
Smoking			
Lifestyle disruptions			
Hospital environment			
Body temperature			
Patient perception of the environment			
Developmental factors			
Genetics factors			
Sleep position			
Pain			
Psychiatric disorders (emotional distress)			

12. Based on your review of the patients in question 11, who is at greatest risk for the nursing diagnosis Sleep pattern: disturbed? For whom are you most concerned regarding a nursing diagnosis of Fatigue? Explain your answers.

→ Now, visit another patient for whom sleep and rest are particularly important—James Story, a 42-year-old man with renal failure. Log our from your current patient and log in to care for Mr. Story at 07:00. Go to his room and click on **Initial Observations**; then assess his Behavior, including each of the assessment subcategories. Afterward, return to the Nurses' Station and open Mr. Story's Chart. Review his Nursing History and his History & Physical.

13. Patients with chronic illness, such as Mr. Story, often meet the criteria for both nursing diagnoses of Sleep pattern: disturbed and Fatigue. In the left column below, list data that support either diagnosis. In the right column, indicate whether each item in your list substantiates a nursing diagnosis of Sleep pattern: disturbed (**S**), Fatigue (**F**), or both (**S and F**).

Supporting Data   **Nursing Diagnosis (S, F, or S and F)**

14. Based on the findings you identified in question 13, you have enough data to write a nursing care plan for either nursing diagnosis (Sleep pattern: disturbed or Fatigue). Select one and identify a goal with individualized nursing interventions for Mr. Story. (*FYI:* For an example of an individualized nursing plan with documentation, refer to the nurse notes for Ms. Emma Weiss and other suggestions under "Evaluation" on p. 936 in your textbook.)

Cognitive-Perceptual Pattern

 Reading Assignment: Managing Pain (Chapter 36)
Managing Confusion (Chapter 39)

Patients: Darlene Martin, Room 613
Elizabeth Washington, Room 604
Maria Ortiz, Room 308
James Story, Room 510

Objectives

1. Assess a patient's need for pain management.
2. Identify the plan for pain management for a patient.
3. Identify risk factors for altered sensory/perceptual function.
4. Identify patients at risk for acute confusion. Plan for prevention. Have a tentative plan to manage acute confusion if it occurs.

Exercise 1—Pain

 This exercise should take approximately 30 minutes to complete.

 Review Table 36-1 (about types of pain) and Table 36-2 (about mechanisms by which drugs relieve pain) on p. 943 in your textbook.

   1. Define the types of pain listed below and on the next page.

Somatic pain

Visceral pain

Referred pain

Neuropathic pain

2. Identify the mechanism by which the following drugs relieve pain.

Nonsteroidal anti-inflammatory drugs (NSAID)

Opiods

Membrane stabilizers, anesthetics, and anticonvulsants

Antidepressants

Noradrenergic agonists

3. Describe the differences among physical dependence, psychological dependence, and pseudoaddiction.

CD-ROM Activity

With *Virtual Clinical Excursions—General Hospital* Disk 2 in your CD-ROM drive, double-click on the **Shortcut to VCE** icon on your computer's desktop. Enter the hospital, click on the elevator, and go to Floor 6. When you arrive on the floor, click on the **Nurses' Station**; then double-click on the **Supervisor's (Login) Computer**. Log in to care for Darlene Martin. Ms. Martin is a 49-year-old patient who was admitted for a total abdominal hysterectomy (TAH) with bilateral salpingo-oophorectomy (BSO). Click on **Patient Records** and select **Chart.** Review the Nursing History.

4. Based on what you learned from Ms. Martin's Nursing History, list examples of the following factors that might affect her pain experience.

Physiologic factors

Cultural and lifestyle factors

Religious factors

Social and environmental factors

→ Return to the Nurses' Station, click on **Patient Records**, and select MAR. Be sure to click on tab **613** to access Ms. Martin's MAR. Review her medication records and begin to plan for her pain management.

5. List five questions you could ask Ms. Martin about her experience with pain, pain medication, and/or her expectations for pain relief.

Exercise 2—Confusion

 This exercise will take approximately 40 minutes to complete.

 Review the causes of and assessment for acute confusion on pp. 1020-1025 in your textbook. You may also want to review general information on acute confusion on pp. 1016-1019.

 6. List the causes of acute confusion.

 7. Of these three Canyon View patients—Ms. Washington, a 63-year-old with a fractured hip who has had an asthma attack and is receiving oxygen; Maria Ortiz, an 8-year-old who has had an asthma attack and is receiving oxygen; and Mr. Story, a 42-year-old who has renal failure, edema, and electrolyte disturbance and is receiving oxygen—which is (are) at risk for acute confusion? Why? Who has the greatest risk? (*Hint:* You may want to review your notes and answers from earlier exercises. If you haven't visited these patients yet, log in to care for each of them at 07:00 and review the Nursing History and the History & Physical sections in their Chart.)

CD-ROM Activity

With *Virtual Clinical Excursions—General Hospital* Disk 2 in your CD-ROM drive, double-click on the **Shortcut to VCE** icon on your computer's desktop. Enter the hospital, click on the elevator, and go to Floor 6. When you arrive on the floor, click on the **Nurses' Station**; then double-click on the **Supervisor's (Login) Computer**. Log in for the 13:00 period of care to visit James Story, who has taken a turn for the worse. If this is the first time you are visiting Mr. Story, open his Chart and read his History & Physical, Nursing History, and Progress Notes to familiarize yourself with his case. Next, access the EPR and analyze Mr. Story's data for any trends, patterns, or sudden changes in his vital signs or other assessment data. Identify priority areas for a focused assessment; then go to his room and perform your assessment. (*Note:* You will record your findings in the table in question 8.)

8. Below, record the findings from your assessment of Mr. Story.

Area of Assessment	Data Collected
Initial Observations	
Vital Signs	
IV	
Wound Condition	
Nutrition	
Behavior	
Head & Neck	
Chest & Back	
GI & GU	
Upper Extremities	
Lower Extremities	

9. Summarize Mr. Story's current neurologic status.

10. List the possible causes of acute confusion that you found in your review of Mr. Story's case. (*Hint:* Be sure you consider his lab results as part of your evidence. If necessary, return to his EPR or to the Laboratory Reports in his Chart for data.)

Self-Perception–Self-Concept Pattern

Reading Assignment: Promoting Self-Concept (Chapter 40)
Managing Anxiety (Chapter 41)
Managing Vulnerability (Chapter 42)

Patients: Darlene Martin, Room 613
Paul Jungerson, Room 602
Julia Parker, Room 608

Objectives

1. Identify teaching strategies that reinforce the elements of self-concept.
2. Recognize actual or potential anxiety in a patient.
3. Plan for strategies to manage or prevent anxiety.
4. Recognize the risk factors for vulnerability.
5. Plan for interventions to empower a vulnerable patient.
6. Recognize the elements of self-concept in an interaction with a patient.

Introduction

In this lesson, you will work with three patients: Darlene Martin, age 49, admitted for a total abdominal hysterectomy and bilateral salpingo-oophorectomy; Paul Jungerson, age 61, who has had a colostomy; and Julia Parker, age 51, who has had a myocardial infarction. As you care for these patients, you will have the opportunity to focus on the importance of issues that relate to self-concept, including body image, personal identity, role performance, and self-esteem.

Exercise 1

 This exercise will take approximately 20 minutes to complete.

 Review about the elements of self-concept on pp. 1036-1039 in your textbook.

 1. In your own words, briefly define *self-concept* and discuss its implications for nursing.

2. In your own words, briefly define *self-esteem*.

3. In addition to self-esteem, self-concept consists of personal identity, role performance, and body image. In your own words, briefly define *personal identity*.

4. In your own words, briefly define *role performance*.

5. In your own words, briefly define *body image*.

6. How do gender differences affect self-esteem? What are the implications for nursing?

CD-ROM Activity

With *Virtual Clinical Excursions—General Hospital* Disk 2 in your CD-ROM drive, double-click on the **Shortcut to VCE** icon on your computer's desktop. Enter the hospital, click on the elevator, and go to Floor 6. When you arrive on the floor, click on the **Nurses' Station**; then double-click on the **Supervisor's (Login) Computer**. Log in to care for Darlene Martin at 11:00. Review her Chart, looking for data to help you assess the concepts you defined in questions 2 through 5 (those terms are listed below). Keep notes of your findings next to each area.

Body image

Self-esteem

Personal identity

Role performance

In your textbook, review pp. 1039-1042 regarding theories of personality development and self-esteem.

7. Consider your own beliefs regarding self-esteem. Do you believe self-esteem is formulated early in life and remains fairly constant, or does it fluctuate with crises and/or transitions? Why do you feel this way?

8. Plot yourself on the self-esteem continuum below by completing steps a, b, and c.

Self-Esteem Continuum

←_____→

Lowest conceivable   Highest conceivable
self-esteem   self-esteem

a. Mark an A to indicate your self-esteem level 1 year before starting nursing school.

b. Mark a B where you are right now.

c. Mark a C where you expect to be after practicing for 1 year as a registered nurse.

9. How do you think your place on the continuum would be affected if you suddenly were hospitalized under the same circumstances as Ms. Parker or Ms. Martin? Why?

10. How do you think your place on the continuum would be affected if you suddenly were hospitalized under the same circumstances as Mr. Jungerson? Why?

11. Regarding self-esteem, what are the implications for nursing?

Review the factors affecting self-concept on pp. 1039-1042 in your textbook.

12. List the factors affecting self-concept.

Review Table 46-1 (Characteristics of People With High Self-Esteem Versus Low Self-Esteem) on p. 1155 of your textbook.

→ If you are currently signed in, go to the Nurses' Station, click on the **Supervisor's (Login) Computer**, and sign out. Then return to the Login Computer and sign in to care for Ms. Parker at 07:00. Go to her room and click on **Initial Observations.** After viewing the interaction between Ms. Parker and the nurse, click on **Behavior** and then click on each of the assessment subcategories: **Signs of Distress, Needs, Support, Understanding,** and **Activity.**

13. Evaluate Ms. Parker's statements in relation to self-concept. How do her statements reflect her self-concept, particularly in regard to self-esteem?

14. For each of the following self-concept issues, list several individualized nursing interventions you believe would be effective in caring for Ms. Parker.

Self-esteem

Personal identity

Role

Body image

→ Return to the Nurses' Station and sign out of the current time period. Once you have logged out, return to the Login Computer and sign in to care for Paul Jungerson at 13:00. Go to his room and click on **Initial Observations**; then conduct a complete Behavior assessment.

15. Evaluate Mr. Jungerson's statements in relation to self-concept. How do his statements reflect his self-concept, particularly in regard to self-esteem?

16. List several individualized nursing interventions you would use in your care for Mr. Jungerson to address the following self-concept issues.

Self-esteem

Personal identity

Role

Body image

Anxiety

Now that you have had the chance to evaluate self-esteem issues for both Ms. Parker and Mr. Jungerson, it is time to begin planning based on nursing diagnosis.

Julia Parker: Through contacts with Ms. Parker, you have identified this nursing diagnosis:
   Anxiety, mild to moderate r/t perceived threats to biological integrity and ego integrity.
In addition, you have developed the following outcome:
   Ms. Parker will report that her anxiety level is tolerable or manageable within 12 hours.

 17. List several nursing interventions to reduce anxiety. (*Hint:* Refer to pp. 1064-1065 in your textbook for suggestions.)

18. Distinguish between the nursing diagnoses Hopelessness and Powerlessness by listing some defining characteristics of each diagnosis below.

Hopelessness   **Powerlessness**

19. If you were caring for a patient who was unable to validate your assessment for Hopelessness, R/O Powerlessness, how would you intervene?

Paul Jungerson: Through contacts with Mr. Jungerson, you have identified this nursing diagnosis:
Powerlessness r/t perceived lack of control over hospital routine and unknown prognosis
In addition, you have developed the following goals:
Mr. Jungerson will verbalize his self-care abilities within 4 hours.
Mr. Jungerson will participate in colostomy care, physical therapy, and problem solving within 24 hours.

 20. List several nursing interventions to reduce vulnerability. Refer to pp. 1086-1087 in your textbook for suggestions.

Role-Relationship Pattern

 Reading Assignment: Managing Functional Limitations (Chapter 43)

Managing Loss (Chapter 44)

Patients: Julia Parker, Room 608
Elizabeth Washington, Room 604
De Olp, Room 310
James Story, Room 512

Objectives

1. Apply the concepts of rehabilitation to discharge planning for selected patients in Canyon View Regional Medical Center.
2. Discuss the implications of various terms associated with functional limitations.
3. Identify the role of members of the rehabilitation team.
4. Apply the concepts of loss to discharge planning for selected patients in Canyon View Regional Medical Center.
5. Compare the nature of the losses experienced by the patients you visit in Canyon View Regional Medical Center.

Exercise 1

 This exercise will take approximately 120 minutes to complete.

 Review concepts of functional limitation on pp. 1092-1093 of your textbook.

1. In your own words, define the following terms (below and on the next page).

Functional limitation

Disability

Impairment

Handicap

Chronic illness

Chronic condition

2. Consider the following personal descriptors (i.e., describing yourself): "I have a functional limitation." "I have a disability." "I have an impairment." "I have a handicap." "I have a chronic illness." "I have a chronic condition."

    a. Which of the descriptors would you consider using to describe yourself (if your condition were such that it applied to you)?

    b. Which would you *never* use?

3. Now consider these descriptors as used by someone else (i.e., someone describing you): "You have a functional limitation." "You have a disability." "You have an impairment." "You have a handicap." "You have a chronic illness." "You have a chronic condition."

    a. Which of these descriptors would you find *least* offensive if they were being used to describe you?

    b. Which would be *most* offensive?

Keep your responses to questions 2 and 3 in mind as you respond to your patients at Canyon View Medical Center and elsewhere.

 Review the section on interdisciplinary teams on pp. 1093-1094 of your textbook.

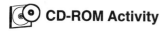 **CD-ROM Activity**

With *Virtual Clinical Excursions—General Hospital* Disk 2 in your CD-ROM drive, double-click on the **Shortcut to VCE** icon on your computer's desktop. Enter the hospital, click on the elevator, and go to Floor 6. When you arrive on the floor, double-click on the **Supervisor's (Login) Computer,** log in to care for Julia Parker at 07:00, and review her Chart.

FYI: Following a myocardial infarction, a patient may be sent to a cardiac rehabilitation program. One purpose is to increase exercise, thus developing collateral circulation to the heart muscle. Another purpose is to make lifestyle changes to decrease the risk for future heart attacks. If she is sent to such a program, Ms. Parker might be exercising on a treadmill, learning about a low-fat diet, getting support to stop smoking, learning stress reduction techniques, and learning about her medications.

4. Below, record any information you found in Ms. Parker's Chart that would help identify her need for rehabilitation and the factors that might affect her rehabilitation.

Need for rehabilitation

Lifestyle factors

Environmental factors

Developmental factors

Cultural/religious factors

Psychosocial factors

Physiologic factors

→ Ms. Parker has a brochure from Canyon View Rehabilitation Center. Apparently overwhelmed, she says, "There seem to be so many people involved in my care here at the hospital and at the rehab facility. What are their responsibilities? Will all these people be involved in my care?"

5. Identify the team members who are currently involved with Ms. Parker and any member(s) who might be included when she enters a rehabilitation program. Address her concerns by informing her in lay terms about the role of each health care provider listed below. Indicate whether or not she can expect to have that type of provider involved in her care.

Rehabilitation nurse

Psychiatrist

Physical therapist

Occupational therapist

Speech therapist

Nutritionist/dietitian

Social worker

Psychologist

Recreational therapist

Prosthetist

Orthotist

Chaplain or spiritual leader of patient's choice

Review the general patient goals of the interdisciplinary rehabilitation team in Box 43-3 on p. 1102. As written, these are team goals for the patient.

 Return to the Nurses' Station and sign out of your care for Ms. Parker, Once you have logged off, return to the Login Computer and sign in to care for Elizabeth Washington at 07:00. Review her Chart as needed to answer questions 6 and 7.

6. Below, record any information you found in Ms. Washington's Chart that would help identify her need for rehabilitation and any factors that might affect her rehabilitation.

Need for rehabilitation

Lifestyle factors

Environmental factors

Developmental factors

Cultural/religious factors

Psychosocial factors

Physiologic factors

7. For each general goal listed below, write expected outcomes that pertain to Ms. Washington. (*Note:* You may combine any that seem repetitive.)

Fostering self-care, self-sufficiency

Encouraging maximal independence level

Maintaining function

Preventing complications

Restoring optimal function

Promoting maximal potential of function

Emphasizing abilities

Adaptation/adjustment

Promoting acceptable quality of life

Maintaining dignity

Reeducation

Community reintegration/reentry

Promoting optimal wellness

8. How would your expected outcomes be different if independence and self-care were not Ms. Washington's prized values?

Review the types of loss on p. 1112 of your textbook. Read the case study of Mike that continues throughout the chapter, especially Box 43-2 on p. 1098.

9. Below, record any information you found in your textbook review that would help identify Mike's losses and any factors that might change the nature of his experience of loss or affect his ability to cope with the losses.

Identification of losses

Developmental factors

Situational factors

Previous experience with loss

Cultural/religious factors

Psychosocial factors

Physiologic factors

→ Return to the Nurses' Station and log out of this period of care. Once you have signed out, go to the elevator, place Disk 1 in your CD-ROM drive, and go to Floor 3. Click on the **Nurses' Station**, access the Login Computer, and sign in to care for De Olp at 07:00. Review her Chart.

10. Record any information you found in De's Chart that would help identify her losses and any factors that might change the nature of her experience of loss or affect her ability to cope with the losses.

Identification of losses

Developmental factors

Situational factors

Previous experience with loss

Cultural/religious factors

Psychosocial factors

Physiologic factors

Once again, return to the Nurses' Station and sign out. Then go to the elevator, place Disk 2 in your CD-ROM drive, and go to Floor 5. Find the Login Computer in the Nurses' Station and sign in to care for James Story at 07:00. Review his Chart.

11. Below, record any information you found in Mr. Story's Chart that would help identify his losses and any factors that might change the nature of his experience of loss or affect his ability to cope with the losses.

Identification of losses

Developmental factors

Situational factors

Previous experience with loss

Cultural/religious factors

Psychosocial factors

Physiologic factors

12. Compare the nature of the losses experienced by Mike and his wife (in the textbook case study), De Olp and her father, Mr. Story and his wife, Ms. Parker, Ms. Martin, and Mr. Jungerson. Address the following factors in your comparison: age of onset of functional limitation, actual loss versus anticipated loss, the effect of the unknowns of prognosis, tangible versus intangible losses, cumulative effects of multiple losses, effects of coping strategies, social support, and a sense of meaning versus meaninglessness.

 To get an idea of the basic tasks of the family, review Table 47-1 (Family Developmental Tasks by Developmental Stage and Age) on p. 1170 in your textbook.

13. Given the variety of the losses discussed in question 12, can you summarize the common outcomes for planning and implementing care? Although these individuals have experienced a wide range of losses, several outcomes are universal. Summarize these common universal outcomes for these patients and/or their family members.

Sexuality-Reproductive Pattern

Reading Assignment: Maintaining Sexual Health (Chapter 45)

Patient: Paul Jungerson, Room 602

Objectives

1. Identify cues to sexuality in a patient.
2. Recognize potential problems in maintaining sexuality
3. Plan for intervention to validate the problem and to assist the patient to maintain an acceptable pattern of sexuality.
4. Recognize traits in yourself that may pose barriers to assisting patients with potential problems in sexuality.

Exercise 1—Sexuality

This exercise will take approximately 45 minutes to complete.

FYI: Here is information that can be shared with your patients about sexuality with an ostomy:
- Your general health, the stress of your illness, or the after-effects of your operation may affect your ability to have intercourse. If you have questions, speak to your stoma care nurse.
- You may resume sexual activity about 6 weeks after your operation, if you wish to. Many people find that their libido (sex drive) decreases. If you do lose interest in sex, don't worry—this isn't unusual. Focus instead on creating a close, loving relationship with your partner. Enjoy activities together and increase your zest for living.
- For a while you may be more tired than usual. If this is a problem, you may want to set aside time for physical intimacy after a period of rest.
- Following your operation you may need to try different sexual positions until you find one that is comfortable for both of you.
- Loss of confidence and a change in the way you see yourself may affect your sexual relationship. Again, this isn't unusual—you may find it helps to talk to your partner about your feelings.
- If you have had your rectum removed, the tissues nearby may be affected. You may find it difficult to have intercourse.
- *For men:* You may have difficulty gaining or maintaining an erection. This can be embarrassing and difficult to discuss. However, your doctor and your stoma care nurse are accustomed to discussing these problems, and even if they are unable to help you themselves, they can refer you to someone who can. Your partner can also be present, if you wish.

- *For women:* Your vagina may be scarred and narrowed. This may make intercourse difficult and painful. You may find it embarrassing to talk about such a personal subject. However, your doctor and your stoma care nurse are accustomed to discussing these problems, and even if they are unable to help you themselves, they can refer you to someone who can. Your partner can also be present, if you wish.

- Remember, enjoyable sex does not have to depend on intercourse alone. There are other ways of showing love and sharing pleasure.

- Living with an ostomy need not interfere with your ability to enjoy an intimate sexual relationship whether it is with a partner in a long-standing relationship or a new partner. You may experience an improved sense of well-being and health after you have recovered from your surgery.

- At first, hesitancy or worry about changes in your desirability and sexual attractiveness is not unusual. Keep in mind that these changes are more likely to be *your* perception than your partner's.

- Another common worry is how to manage the pouch during intercourse. Concerns include odor, the presence of stool in the bag, and the perception that the pouch and stoma will be unsightly to your partner. It might take a little planning. You can check ahead of time to be sure the bag is empty; you may also cover the bag with underwear or a cummerbund. Some women choose to wear crotchless underwear.

- If you are using a two-piece system, mini-pouches or stoma caps are available to make the appliance more discreet; you can switch to this before engaging in sexual activity. Smaller pouches and caps have a limited capacity and should not be worn for extended periods of time. If wearing your regular pouch, try to empty the pouch before beginning sexual relations. Some people like to secure the pouch against their skin, to minimize its movement and lessen any "rustly" noises; this can be done simply with tape or more creatively with things such as cummerbunds or crotchless underwear.

- Open communication with your partner before getting into a sexual situation will help dissipate discomfort and the element of surprise. Share your experience with your partner and dispel any concerns or worries. Comfort and confidence will come with time. Being sensitive to your partner's and your personal needs is no more crucial now than in any other previous sexual experience.

- Although sexual activity will not hurt your stoma, some positions may be more comfortable than others. Maintaining a sense of humor throughout your experiences and experiments will also help with the transition.

- If you are entering a new relationship and it is progressing toward intimacy, disclosure well in advance of sexual activity is helpful to make the relationship work for both of you. Although the amount of information you decide to share about your illness is a personal choice, you may want to start the conversation with a comment such as this: "I had an illness that required surgery on my bowel; I needed to have my bowel diverted to the outside and now I have an ostomy. The surgery has allowed me to feel healthy again."

 1. List five factors that might need to be addressed or managed when you are working with a patient who has concerns about sexual issues related to a medical or surgical problem.

    a.

    b.

    c.

    d.

    e.

    f.

CD-ROM Activity

With *Virtual Clinical Excursions—General Hospital* Disk 2 in your CD-ROM drive, double-click on the **Shortcut to VCE** icon on your computer's desktop. Enter the hospital, click on the elevator, and go to Floor 6. When you arrive on the floor, click on the **Nurses' Station**; then double-click on the **Supervisor's (Login) Computer**. Log in to care for Paul Jungerson at 09:00. Open his Chart and review the Nursing History and the History & Physical.

2. Use the table below to record data from your Chart review relevant to Mr. Jungerson's sexuality. Also formulate questions that you would like to ask him concerning this issue.

Factors Affecting Sexuality	Data About Mr. Jungerson/Questions to Ask
Developmental issues	
Physiologic factors	
Cultural/lifestyle factors	

3. Provide a definition for each of the following nursing diagnoses.

Ineffective sexuality pattern

Sexual dysfunction

4. Which nursing diagnosis would you select for Mr. Jungerson? Why?

5. List the steps of the PLISSIT Model and give a brief description of each.

6. Imagine that you are going to provide information to Mr. Jungerson about sexual health after a colostomy. How would you approach the issues and related problems?

Coping–Stress Tolerance Pattern

 Reading Assignment: Supporting Stress Tolerance and Coping (Chapter 46)
Supporting Family Coping (Chapter 47)

Patients: De Olp, Room 310
James Story, Room 512

Objectives

1. Identify the effective and ineffective coping behaviors of a patient.
2. Identify the tasks of a caregiver for a patient with chronic illness.
3. Identify the risk for caregiver role strain for a patient with chronic illness.
4. Identify health-teaching needs for the parents of a school-age child.
5. Identify the strengths and weakness of a family to manage a health problem.

Exercise 1—Coping-Stress Tolerance

 This exercise will take approximately 30 minutes to complete.

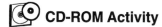 Review the concepts of stress, concepts of coping, and factors affecting stress tolerance, on pp. 1153-1157 of your textbook.

CD-ROM Activity

With *Virtual Clinical Excursions—General Hospital* Disk 2 in your CD-ROM drive, double-click on the **Shortcut to VCE** icon on your computer's desktop. Enter the hospital, click on the elevator, and go to Floor 5. When you arrive on the floor, click on the **Nurses' Station**; then double-click on the **Supervisor's (Login) Computer**. Log in to care for Mr. Story at 09:00 and review his Chart. Next, go to his room and observe the Behavior assessment.

Consider the following scenario and interaction as your answer questions 1 through 4:

You honor Mr. Story's request and call his wife, requesting her to come visit when she can. After she arrives, you decide to offer her assistance and ask her, "By the way, Mrs. Story, do you have what you need?" She answers without hesitation, "Yes, I do." Then you ask her, "How do you cope?" She responds, "Jim always says, 'Coping is not optional.'" You follow up with another question: "Are your coping strategies effective?" After pausing to think for a moment, Mrs. Story asks you, "How can you tell the difference?"

1. Describe an example of adaptive and maladaptive coping for Mr. Story.

2. Mrs. Story continues her conversation with you. She says, "Jim has told me that he used to deny and rationalize a lot—that these were his favorite defense mechanisms. How do defense mechanisms fit with coping?" Write a response to Mrs. Story's question.

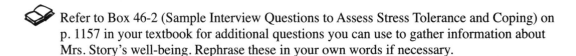 Refer to Box 46-2 (Sample Interview Questions to Assess Stress Tolerance and Coping) on p. 1157 in your textbook for additional questions you can use to gather information about Mrs. Story's well-being. Rephrase these in your own words if necessary.

3. List two challenges to coping skills.

4. List two factors affecting stress tolerance.

Exercise 2—Family Coping

 This exercise will take approximately 30 minutes to complete.

 Review "Concepts of Family," "Factors Affecting Family Coping," and "Family Assessment," on pp. 1167-1179 of your textbook. Then review Box 46-2 (Sample Interview Questions to Assess Stress Tolerance and Coping) on p. 1157.

FYI: In order to begin your stress and coping assessment for the family, it may be most helpful for you to begin by assessing one particular patient or family member for individual stress tolerance and coping. It may be less threatening for a family member to share about himself of herself before disclosing family information.

Review Table 47-2 (Family Assessment Criteria) on p. 1176 in your textbook.

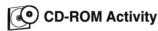 **CD-ROM Activity**

If you are not currently logged in for Mr. Story, log in now for the 09:00-10:29 period of care. Consider the logistics of completing the family assessment for Mr. and Mrs. Story. If necessary, visit the patient in his room or review his records to answer questions 5 and 6.

5. Below, record any information you found in each of the categories of family assessment criteria. Which information were you unable to obtain? Consider the needs of both Mr. and Mrs. Story. List some strategies that you could use to gather this additional information. Which answers could be obtained by interview? Which questions require assessment of the family's interactions over time?

Physical needs

Protection

Health promotion

Communication

6. Can you identify other methods to obtain the information that you could not get from visiting Mr. Story at this time?

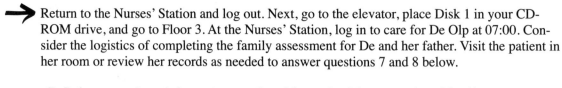 Return to the Nurses' Station and log out. Next, go to the elevator, place Disk 1 in your CD-ROM drive, and go to Floor 3. At the Nurses' Station, log in to care for De Olp at 07:00. Consider the logistics of completing the family assessment for De and her father. Visit the patient in her room or review her records as needed to answer questions 7 and 8 below.

7. Below, record any information you found for each of the categories of family assessment criteria. Which information were you unable to obtain? Consider the needs of both De and her father. List some strategies below that you could use to gather this additional information. Which answers could be obtained by interview? Which questions require assessment of the family's interactions over time?

Physical needs

Protection

Health promotion

Communication

8. Can you identify other methods to obtain the information that you could not get from visiting De and her father at this time?

9. Would you want to interview the family members together or separately? Explain.

10. What issues can you predict may get in the way of your obtaining accurate information? (*Hint:* Review the questions in Table 47-2 and consider why *you* might not give a truthful answer.)

11. If you were going to follow the family after discharge, what other methods would you use to obtain answers to the questions in Table 47-2?

Value-Belief Pattern

Objectives

1. Identify actual or potential signs of a spiritual need.
2. Plan interventions to meet an actual or potential spiritual need or to support spiritual practices.

Exercise 1: Spirituality

 This exercise will take approximately 45 minutes to complete.

 Read "Concepts of Spirituality" on pp. 1187-1192 in your textbook.

1. In your own words, briefly define *spirituality*.

2. Briefly summarize Germere's findings regarding spirituality and health.

3. Describe the importance of spiritual well-being to health.

4. What characterizes spiritual health? Why is it important to nursing?

5. What barriers exist for providing spiritual nursing care?

6. Now assess yourself. What barriers exist for you in providing spiritual nursing care?

7. Many of your patients are likely to be older adults. How would you characterize the spiritual needs of older adults?

8. What specific questions can you ask in order to assess someone's spiritual well-being?

9. In your own words, list nursing interventions that assess spiritual well-being and address spiritual distress.

CD-ROM Activity

With *Virtual Clinical Excursions—General Hospital* Disk 2 in your CD-ROM drive, double-click on the **Shortcut to VCE** icon on your computer's desktop. Enter the hospital, click on the elevator, and go to Floor 3. When you arrive on the floor, click on the **Nurses' Station**; then double-click on the **Supervisor's (Login) Computer**. Sign in to visit Maria Ortiz at 07:00. Now return to the Nurses' Station, click on **Patient Records**, and select **Chart**. Review Maria's Chart for data related to her spirituality.

10. Record your findings regarding Maria's spirituality below.

Religion

Religious practices

Relationship to the universe

Elements that could produce doubts in faith

Relationship with others

Additional data you might seek in your conversations with the patient

As you care for Maria and collect data regarding her spirituality, you elicit the following statements from her:

- "I made my first Communion last year."
- "My mother and I usually meet the rest of my family at Mass each Sunday, and then we go to one of their houses to visit."
- "I believe we'll all go to heaven, no matter what religion we are on Earth."
- "I don't understand why God would make me sick, but my mother and I believe He has a plan that maybe I'll understand as I get older."
- "I get scared when I have asthma attacks, but it helps me to think that even if I die, I'll go to heaven."
- "I feel connected with my mother and the rest of my family . . . and to the other people in church when I'm there."

11. Based on the above statements, what is your assessment of Maria's spiritual well-being? What nursing interventions are indicated?

Return to the Nurses' Station and sign out of this period of care. Then go to the elevator, place Disk 2 in your CD-ROM drive, and go to Floor 6. At the Nurses' Station, log in to care for Paul Jungerson at 07:00. Review Mr. Jungerson's Chart for data regarding his spirituality.

 12. Record your findings regarding Mr. Jungerson's spirituality below.

Religion

Religious practices

Relationship to the universe

Elements that could produce doubts in faith

Relationship with others

Additional data you might seek in your conversations with the patent

As you care for Mr. Jungerson and collect data regarding his spirituality, you elicit the following statements from him:

- "At times, it's hard to believe that my wife died first. She was a good person . . . I wish God had taken me first."
- "I often find myself wondering, 'What's the point of it all?'"
- "With my son, there's still a lot that is unresolved. It will probably never be different . . . I really don't want to talk about it."

13. Based on the above statements, what is your assessment of Mr. Jungerson's spiritual well-being? What nursing interventions are indicated?

Notes:

Notes:

Notes:

Notes:

Notes:

Notes:

Notes:

Notes:

Notes: